Chronic HCV Infection: Clinical Advances and Eradication Perspectives

Chronic HCV Infection: Clinical Advances and Eradication Perspectives

Editors

Maria Carla Liberto
Nadia Marascio

MDPI • Basel • Beijing • Wuhan • Barcelona • Belgrade • Manchester • Tokyo • Cluj • Tianjin

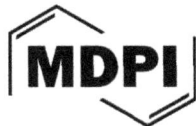

Editors
Maria Carla Liberto
Department of Health Sciences,
Unit of Clinical Microbiology,
"Magna Graecia" University
Italy

Nadia Marascio
Department of Health Sciences,
Unit of Clinical Microbiology,
"Magna Graecia" University
Italy

Editorial Office
MDPI
St. Alban-Anlage 66
4052 Basel, Switzerland

This is a reprint of articles from the Special Issue published online in the open access journal *Journal of Clinical Medicine* (ISSN 2077-0383) (available at: https://www.mdpi.com/journal/jcm/special_issues/Chronic_HCV_Infection).

For citation purposes, cite each article independently as indicated on the article page online and as indicated below:

LastName, A.A.; LastName, B.B.; LastName, C.C. Article Title. *Journal Name* **Year**, *Volume Number*, Page Range.

ISBN 978-3-0365-3361-2 (Hbk)
ISBN 978-3-0365-3362-9 (PDF)

© 2022 by the authors. Articles in this book are Open Access and distributed under the Creative Commons Attribution (CC BY) license, which allows users to download, copy and build upon published articles, as long as the author and publisher are properly credited, which ensures maximum dissemination and a wider impact of our publications.

The book as a whole is distributed by MDPI under the terms and conditions of the Creative Commons license CC BY-NC-ND.

Contents

Maria Carla Liberto and Nadia Marascio
Special Issue "Chronic HCV Infection: Clinical Advances and Eradication Perspectives"
Reprinted from: *J. Clin. Med.* 2022, 11, 359, doi:10.3390/jcm11020359 1

Jur-Shan Cheng, Yu-Sheng Lin, Jing-Hong Hu, Ming-Yu Chang, Hsin-Ping Ku, Rong-Nan Chien and Ming-Ling Chang
Impact of Interferon-Based Therapy on Hepatitis C-Associated Rheumatic Diseases: A Nationwide Population-Based Cohort Study
Reprinted from: *J. Clin. Med.* 2021, 10, 817, doi:10.3390/jcm10040817 5

Nadia Marascio, Angela Costantino, Stefania Taffon, Alessandra Lo Presti, Michele Equestre, Roberto Bruni, Giulio Pisani, Giorgio Settimo Barreca, Angela Quirino, Enrico Maria Trecarichi, Chiara Costa, Maria Mazzitelli, Francesca Serapide, Giovanni Matera, Carlo Torti, Maria Carla Liberto and Anna Rita Ciccaglione
Phylogenetic and Molecular Analyses of More Prevalent HCV1b Subtype in the Calabria Region, Southern Italy
Reprinted from: *J. Clin. Med.* 2021, 10, 1655, doi:10.3390/jcm10081655 19

Mira Florea, Teodora Serban, George Razvan Tirpe, Alexandru Tirpe and Monica Lupsor-Platon
Noninvasive Assessment of Hepatitis C Virus Infected Patients Using Vibration-Controlled Transient Elastography
Reprinted from: *J. Clin. Med.* 2021, 10, 2575, doi:10.3390/jcm10122575 31

Dorota Zarębska-Michaluk, Jerzy Jaroszewicz, Anna Parfieniuk-Kowerda, Ewa Janczewska, Dorota Dybowska, Małgorzata Pawłowska, Waldemar Halota, Włodzimierz Mazur, Beata Lorenc, Justyna Janocha-Litwin, Krzysztof Simon, Anna Piekarska, Hanna Berak, Jakub Klapaczyński, Piotr Stępień, Barbara Sobala-Szczygieł, Jolanta Citko, Łukasz Socha, Magdalena Tudrujek-Zdunek, Krzysztof Tomasiewicz, Marek Sitko, Beata Dobracka, Rafał Krygier, Jolanta Białkowska-Warzecha, Łukasz Laurans and Robert Flisiak
Effectiveness and Safety of Pangenotypic Regimens in the Most Difficult to Treat Population of Genotype 3 HCV Infected Cirrhotics
Reprinted from: *J. Clin. Med.* 2021, 10, 3280, doi:10.3390/jcm10153280 51

Maria Pokorska-Śpiewak, Anna Dobrzeniecka, Małgorzata Aniszewska and Magdalena Marczyńska
Real-Life Experience with Ledipasvir/Sofosbuvir for the Treatment of Chronic Hepatitis C Virus Infection with Genotypes 1 and 4 in Children Aged 12 to 17 Years—Results of the POLAC Project
Reprinted from: *J. Clin. Med.* 2021, 10, 4176, doi:10.3390/jcm10184176 65

Marleen van Dijk, Sylvia M. Brakenhoff, Cas J. Isfordink, Wei-Han Cheng, Hans Blokzijl, Greet Boland, Anthonius S. M. Dofferhoff, Bart van Hoek, Cees van Nieuwkoop, Milan J. Sonneveld, Marc van der Valk, Joost P. H. Drenth and Robert J. de Knegt
The Netherlands Is on Track to Meet the World Health Organization Hepatitis C Elimination Targets by 2030
Reprinted from: *J. Clin. Med.* 2021, 10, 4562, doi:10.3390/jcm10194562 75

Bianca Granozzi, Viola Guardigni, Lorenzo Badia, Elena Rosselli Del Turco, Alberto Zuppiroli, Beatrice Tazza, Pietro Malosso, Stefano Pieralli, Pierluigi Viale and Gabriella Verucchi
Out-of-Hospital Treatment of Hepatitis C Increases Retention in Care among People Who Inject Drugs and Homeless Persons: An Observational Study
Reprinted from: *J. Clin. Med.* **2021**, *10*, 4955, doi:10.3390/jcm10214955 . . . . **87**

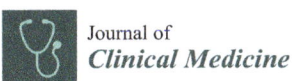

Editorial

Special Issue "Chronic HCV Infection: Clinical Advances and Eradication Perspectives"

Maria Carla Liberto * and Nadia Marascio *

Unit of Microbiology, Department of Health Sciences, "Magna Graecia" University, 88100 Catanzaro, Italy
* Correspondence: mliberto@unicz.it (M.C.L.); nadiamarascio@gmail.com (N.M.)

Citation: Liberto, M.C.; Marascio, N. Special Issue "Chronic HCV Infection: Clinical Advances and Eradication Perspectives". *J. Clin. Med.* **2022**, *11*, 359. https://doi.org/10.3390/jcm11020359

Received: 10 January 2022
Accepted: 11 January 2022
Published: 12 January 2022

Publisher's Note: MDPI stays neutral with regard to jurisdictional claims in published maps and institutional affiliations.

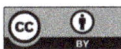

Copyright: © 2022 by the authors. Licensee MDPI, Basel, Switzerland. This article is an open access article distributed under the terms and conditions of the Creative Commons Attribution (CC BY) license (https:// creativecommons.org/licenses/by/ 4.0/).

The latest report of global hepatitis estimated 58 million people with Hepatitis C virus (HCV) chronic disease and 1.5 million newly infected subjects per year [1]. In 2016, the World Health Organization (WHO) proposed a plan to reduce new infections and related deaths by 2030 [1]. However, the current severe acute respiratory syndrome coronavirus 2 (SARS-CoV-2) pandemic has determined a reallocation of public health resources, with a consequent delay in the hepatitis elimination program, already documented in Egypt and Italy [2]. In this Special Issue, we discuss the HCV eradication perspective related to the global situation before and during the ongoing pandemic. Direct-acting antiviral (DAA) agent efficacy, diagnostic methods and screening policy have all been evaluated via seven papers, six original articles and one review.

The keywords with respect to the WHO plan are timely diagnosis and effective treatment for all infected individuals. The homeless and people who inject drugs (PWID), mono- or co-infected with HCV, have poor access to screening tests, medical care and showed a high reinfection rate after sustained viral response (SVR) [3]. In Italy, between January and June 2019, an observational study linked to these specific risk groups was carried out. The out-of-hospital model was able to guarantee better adherence to antiviral treatment and prevention of new HCV infections compared to the in-hospital model. Standard approaches need to be integrated with new healthcare strategies to achieve elimination of infection in the general, as well as in the neglected population [4].

Several studies: Using mathematical methods, an attempt was made to trace HCV elimination in different countries, highlighting tailored national interventions to achieve this goal [5]. Taking into account overall population, viremic patients, new diagnoses and other parameters to perform Model Base-Case, van Dijk and co-workers reported two main scenarios in the Netherlands. In the Status Quo scenario, the HCV target was set for 2027, while in the Gradual Decline scenario, for 2032. Interestingly, COVID-19 scenarios showed an increased number of decompensated cirrhosis and hepatocellular carcinoma (HCC) without significant delay in HCV eradication [6]. HCV infection is diagnosed by serological and molecular tests, while treatment and prognosis are related to liver damage and comorbidities [7,8]. Even if liver biopsy is the gold standard, conventional ultrasonography (US) and vibration-controlled transient elastography (VCTE) are noninvasive and cost-efficient methods currently adopted to measure fibrosis and steatosis progression. Florea et al. believed that performance of VCTE was superior to the conventional US technique due to the high negative predictive value and greater specificity. In the near future, VCTE could be very useful for risk prediction of HCC in HCV positive patients [9]. HCV is associated with hepatic and extra-hepatic illness, such as rheumatic diseases, which can be alleviated after antiviral therapy [8,10]. Cheng and coauthors, conducting a nationwide population study, reported how interferon (IFN) therapy did not mitigate rheumatic disease risk. On the contrary, the IFN-free treatment effect after SVR needs to be further investigated [10].

Pan-genotypic therapy is used to treat HCV infected people independently of the genotype resistance test [11]. Nevertheless, real life data show that DAA efficacy can be influenced by resistance-associated substitutions (RASs) carried by target genomic regions.

Between 2015 and 2016, we enrolled 41 HCV1b positive patients who reported surgical intervention, unsafe use of glass syringes, and dental treatment as risk factors. We analyzed the HCV1b viral isolates to evaluate the presence of RASs in NS5A and NS5B amplicons. In particular, in 36.5% of NS5B sequences, L159F was carried alone and in 19.5% was found in combination with C316N, both associated with lower response to sofosbuvir (SOF). On the other hand, three NS5A sequences displayed the Y93H RAS currently responsible for many DAA regimen failures [12]. In 2017, the ledipasvir (LDV)/SOF combination was approved by the European Medical Agency (EMA) and the Food and Drug Administration (FDA) to cure children 12–17 years old. Pokorska-Śpiewak et al. reported efficacy and safety of LDV/SOF therapy in adolescents with HCV chronic diseases infected by HCV1 or HCV4. The study had limitations on data collection due to the SARS-CoV-2 pandemic [13]. These results are in line with our previously published paper. Two HCV4 pediatric patients achieved SVR, although viral isolates carried both the L28M and M31L NS5A RASs [14]. Despite the high SVR rate in pan-genotypic regimens, at present HCV3 is the most difficult-to-treat genotype, especially in cirrhotic and DAA-treated patients. However, real-world data reported by Zarębska-Michaluk and co-authors showed the higher effectiveness of glecaprevir/pibrentasvir (96%) compared to SOF/velpatasvir (VEL) (93%) and to SOF/VEL + ribavirin (79%) regimens [15].

Funding: This research received no external funding.

Acknowledgments: We would like to thank the authors for their valuable scientific papers, reviewers for their improvement suggestions and the *JCM* Editorial Office for their professional support.

Conflicts of Interest: The authors declare no conflict of interest.

References

1. World Health Organization (WHO). Available online: https://www.who.int (accessed on 2 January 2022).
2. Blach, S.; Kondili, L.A.; Aghemo, A.; Cai, Z.; Dugan, E.; Estes, C.; Gamkrelidze, I.; Ma, S.; Pawlotsky, J.M.; Razavi-Shearer, D.; et al. Impact of COVID-19 on global HCV elimination efforts. *J. Hepatol.* **2021**, *74*, 31–36. [CrossRef] [PubMed]
3. Remy, A.-J.; Bouchkira, H. Successful Cascade of Care and Cure HCV in 5382 Drugs Users: How Increase HCV Treatment by Outreach Care, Since Screening to Treatment. *J. Dig. Disord. Diagn.* **2019**, *1*, 27–35. [CrossRef]
4. Granozzi, B.; Guardigni, V.; Badiam, L.; Rosselli Del Turco, E.; Zuppiroli, A.; Tazza, B.; Malosso, P.; Pieralli, S.; Viale, P.; Verucchi, G. Out-of-Hospital Treatment of Hepatitis C Increases Retention in Care among People Who Inject Drugs and Homeless Persons: An Observational Study. *J. Clin. Med.* **2021**, *10*, 4955. [CrossRef] [PubMed]
5. Gamkrelidze, I.; Pawlotsky, J.; Lazarus, J.V.; Feld, J.J.; Zeuzem, S.; Bao, Y.; dos Santos, A.G.P.; Gonzalez, Y.S.; Razavi, H. Progress towards hepatitis C virus elimination in high-income countries: An updated analysis. *Liver Int.* **2021**, *41*, 456–463. [CrossRef] [PubMed]
6. van Dijk, M.; Brakenhoff, S.M.; Isfordink, C.J.; Cheng, W.H.; Blokzijl, H.; Boland, G.; Dofferhoff, A.S.M.; van Hoek, B.; van Nieuwkoop, C.; Sonneveld, M.J.; et al. The Netherlands Is on Track to Meet the World Health Organization Hepatitis C Elimination Targets by 2030. *J. Clin. Med.* **2021**, *10*, 4562. [CrossRef] [PubMed]
7. Morozov, V.A.; Lagaye, S. Hepatitis C virus: Morphogenesis, infection and therapy. *World J. Hepatol.* **2018**, *10*, 186–212. [CrossRef] [PubMed]
8. Sebastiani, M.; Giuggioli, D.; Colaci, M.; Fallahi, P.; Gragnani, L.; Antonelli, A.; Zignego, A.L.; Ferri, C. HCV-related rheumatic manifestations and therapeutic strategies. *Curr. Drug Targets* **2017**, *18*, 803–810. [CrossRef] [PubMed]
9. Florea, M.; Serban, T.; Tirpe, G.R.; Tirpe, A.; Lupsor-Platon, M. Noninvasive Assessment of Hepatitis C Virus Infected Patients Using Vibration-Controlled Transient Elastography. *J. Clin. Med.* **2021**, *10*, 2575. [CrossRef] [PubMed]
10. Cheng, J.S.; Lin, Y.S.; Hu, J.H.; Chang, M.Y.; Ku, H.P.; Chien, R.N.; Chang, M.L. Impact of Interferon-Based Therapy on Hepatitis C-Associated Rheumatic Diseases: A Nationwide Population-Based Cohort Study. *J. Clin. Med.* **2021**, *10*, 817. [CrossRef] [PubMed]
11. European Association for the Study of the Liver. EASL Recommendations on Treatment of Hepatitis C 2020. *J. Hepatol.* **2020**, *73*, 1170–1218.
12. Marascio, N.; Costantino, A.; Taffon, S.; Lo Presti, A.; Equestre, M.; Bruni, R.; Pisani, G.; Barreca, G.S.; Quirino, A.; Trecarichi, E.M.; et al. Phylogenetic and Molecular Analyses of More Prevalent HCV1b Subtype in the Calabria Region, Southern Italy. *J. Clin. Med.* **2021**, *10*, 1655. [CrossRef] [PubMed]
13. Pokorska-Śpiewak, M.; Dobrzeniecka, A.; Aniszewska, M.; Marczyńska, M. Real-Life Experience with Ledipasvir/Sofosbuvir for the Treatment of Chronic Hepatitis C Virus Infection with Genotypes 1 and 4 in Children Aged 12 to 17 Years-Results of the POLAC Project. *J. Clin. Med.* **2021**, *10*, 4176. [CrossRef] [PubMed]

14. Marascio, N.; Mazzitelli, M.; Pavia, G.; Giancotti, A.; Barreca, G.S.; Costa, C.; Pisani, V.; Greco, G.; Serapide, F.; Trecarichi, E.M.; et al. Clinical, Virological Characteristics, and Outcomes of Treatment with Sofosbuvir/Ledipasvir in Two Pediatric Patients Infected by HCV Genotype 4. *Cells* **2019**, *8*, 416. [CrossRef] [PubMed]
15. Zarębska-Michaluk, D.; Jaroszewicz, J.; Parfieniuk-Kowerda, A.; Janczewska, E.; Dybowska, D.; Pawłowska, M.; Halota, W.; Mazur, W.; Lorenc, B.; Janocha-Litwin, J.; et al. Effectiveness and Safety of Pangenotypic Regimens in the Most Difficult to Treat Population of Genotype 3 HCV Infected Cirrhotics. *J. Clin. Med.* **2021**, *10*, 3280. [CrossRef] [PubMed]

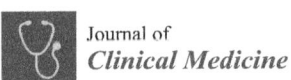

Article

Impact of Interferon-Based Therapy on Hepatitis C-Associated Rheumatic Diseases: A Nationwide Population-Based Cohort Study

Jur-Shan Cheng [1,2], Yu-Sheng Lin [3,4], Jing-Hong Hu [5], Ming-Yu Chang [6,7,8], Hsin-Ping Ku [2], Rong-Nan Chien [8,9] and Ming-Ling Chang [8,9,*]

1. Clinical Informatics and Medical Statistics Research Center, College of Medicine, Chang Gung University, Taoyuan 333323, Taiwan; jscheng@mail.cgu.edu.tw
2. Department of Emergency Medicine, Chang Gung Memorial Hospital, Keelung 20401, Taiwan; find94132@yahoo.com
3. Department of Cardiology, Chang Gung Memorial Hospital, Taoyuan 333423, Taiwan; ma3958@gmail.com
4. Healthcare Center, Chang Gung Memorial Hospital, Taoyuan 333423, Taiwan
5. Department of Internal Medicine, Chang Gung Memorial Hospital, Yunlin 63862, Taiwan; a3237184@gmail.co
6. Division of Pediatric Neurologic Medicine, Chang Gung Children's Hospital, Taoyuan 333423, Taiwan; p123073@gmail.com
7. Division of Pediatrics, Chang Gung Memorial Hospital, Keelung 20401, Taiwan
8. Department of Medicine, College of Medicine, Chang Gung University, Taoyuan 333423, Taiwan; ronald@cgmh.org.tw
9. Division of Gastroenterology, Department of Gastroenterology and Hepatology, Chang Gung Memorial Hospital, Taoyuan 333423, Taiwan
* Correspondence: mlchang8210@gmail.com; Tel.: +886-3-3281200-8102; Fax: +886-3-3272236

Abstract: Whether hepatitis C virus (HCV) infection-associated risk of rheumatic diseases is reversed by anti-HCV therapy remain elusive. A nationwide population-based cohort study of the Taiwan National Health Insurance Research Database was conducted. Of 19,298,735 subjects, 3 cohorts (1:4:4, propensity score-matched), including HCV-treated (6919 HCV-infected subjects with interferon and ribavirin therapy ≥ 6 months), HCV-untreated (n = 27,676) and HCV-uninfected (n = 27,676) cohorts, were enrolled and followed (2003–2015). The HCV-uninfected cohort had the lowest cumulative incidence of rheumatic diseases (95% confidence interval (CI): 8.416–10.734%), while HCV-treated (12.417–17.704%) and HCV-untreated (13.585–16.479%) cohorts showed no difference in the cumulative incidences. Multivariate analyses showed that HCV infection (95% CI hazard ratio (HR): 1.54–1.765), female sex (1.57–1.789), age ≥ 49 years (1.091–1.257), Charlson comorbidity index ≥ 1 (1.075–1.245), liver cirrhosis (0.655–0.916), chronic obstruction pulmonary disease (1.130–1.360), end-stage renal disease (0.553–0.98), diabetes mellitus (0.834–0.991) and dyslipidemia (1.102–1.304) were associated with incident rheumatic diseases. Among the 3 cohorts, the untreated cohort had the highest cumulative incidence of overall mortality, while the treated and un-infected cohorts had indifferent mortalities. Conclusions: HCV infection, baseline demographics and comorbidities were associated with rheumatic diseases. Although HCV-associated risk of rheumatic diseases might not be reversed by interferon-based therapy, which reduced the overall mortality in HCV-infected patients.

Keywords: HCV; rheumatic; interferon; mortality

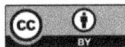

1. Introduction

Hepatitis C virus (HCV) is a human pathogen responsible for acute and chronic liver disease that infects an estimated 150 million individuals worldwide [1]. In addition to hepatic complications including cirrhosis and hepatocellular carcinoma, HCV may cause many extrahepatic complications such as diabetes mellitus (DM), hypolipidemia, cardiovascular events [1], and rheumatic diseases [2]. HCV is both hepatotropic and lymphotropic [3]. HCV lymphotropism represents the most important step in the pathogenesis of virus-related immunological diseases [4], especially rheumatic diseases. Rheumatologic extrahepatic manifestations are observed in 2% to 38% of HCV-infected patients [5], and this variability is attributed to the various geographic region and design of the studies [6–8]. Moreover, HCV antibodies were found in 18.5% among patients admitted to the rheumatology ward [9], being higher than the estimated global prevalence (2.2–2.8%) of HCV infection [10]. The Hispanoamerican Study Group of Autoimmune Manifestations associated with Hepatitis C Virus (HISPAMEC) Registry showed that the systemic autoimmune diseases most associated with chronic HCV infection were Sjogren syndrome (SS), rheumatoid arthritis (RA) and systemic lupus erythematosus (SLE) [11]. Specifically, the co-prevalence of HCV and SS ranged from 49% [12] to 80% [13], HCV infection was found in 13% of a large series of Spanish patients with SS [14], and sicca symptoms were reported in 11% of French HCV patients [15]. HCV infection was also associated with increased RA risks [16,17], and the pooled prevalence of RA was 4.5% (0.6–25.7%) of chronic HCV-infected patients in East Asia [2]. Moreover, the prevalence of HCV infection among SLE patients was found to be 10% [18].

The combination of pegylated interferon (Peg-IFN) and ribavirin has provided a "cure" for a considerable proportion of patients with chronic hepatitis C infection (CHC), particularly in patients with a favorable interferon λ 3 (IFNL3) genotype [1]. These cure rates were further improved by replacing interferon-based therapy with potent, direct-acting antiviral agents (DAAs) [1], and the sustained virological response rate (SVR) to DAA in HCV-infected patients is approaching 100% [19]. However, some HCV-associated complications such as cardiometabolic and oncogenic events cannot be reversed, even after viral clearance [1,20,21]. Whether the HCV-associated risk of rheumatic diseases can be attenuated after the completion of anti-HCV therapy thus is still a crucial issue of public health in the era of DAA to eradicate HCV infection but remains elusive.

Accordingly, we conducted a nationwide population-based cohort study in Taiwan, where HCV infection is rampant [22]. The impacts of HCV infection and anti-HCV therapy on the risk of rheumatic diseases were investigated by comparing the cumulative incidences of rheumatic diseases and of the overall mortalities among HCV-infected subjects with and without anti-HCV therapy and the subjects without HCV infection, based on data from the Taiwan National Health Insurance Research Database (TNHIRD). This database provides medical information of the nationwide population, which comprises 26,573,661 individuals.

2. Methods
2.1. TNHIRD Samples and Measurements

This population-based retrospective cohort study used nation-level data, including the National Health Insurance (NHI) administrative database, the Cancer Registry Database, and the Death Registry Database of Taiwan. The mandatory, single-payer NHI program provides comprehensive coverage including ambulatory care, hospital services, laboratory tests, and prescription drugs. Over 99% of the population is enrolled in the program and approximately 90% of the healthcare organizations are contracted with NHI Administration. Given that Taiwan is a hyperendemic area for hepatitis B virus (HBV) infection, which is highly oncogenic, causes many hepatic complications and prominently biases the phenotype of HCV infection [23], the subjects diagnosed with HBV infection in the observation period (2003–2015), or with any baseline rheumatic diseases including RA (International Classification of Disease, Ninth. Revision, Clinical Modification (ICD-9-CM) code (714)), ankylosing spondylitis (ICD-9-CM code (720)) [24], psoriatic arthopathy (ICD-9-CM code (696.0)), sicca syndrome (also called SS) (ICD-9-CM code (710.2)), systemic sclerosis (ICD-9-CM code (710.1)), SLE (ICD-9-CM code (710.0)), Behcet's syndrome (ICD-9-CM code (136.1)) [25], Raynaud's syndrome (ICD-9-CM code (443.0)), polyarteritis nodosa and allied conditions (ICD-9-CM code (446)) [26], and psoriasis (ICD-9-CM code (696.X)) [27] or mortality occurred prior to 6 months after completing anti-HCV treatment (the baseline), when it is the time to ensure therapeutic response, were excluded.

The HCV-treated cohort included subjects who had a HCV RNA test and received ribavirin and pegylated interferon (Peg-IFN) in 2003–2015. Their first HCV test was assumed to be the index date of diagnosis. The baseline for the HCV-treated cohort was the date of 6 months after completing the combination therapy. Untreated HCV-infected patients were those who had been examined for HCV infection (HCV antibody or HCV RNA test) (their first HCV test was the index date), were diagnosed with HCV (The International Classification of Diseases, Ninth Revision, Clinical Modification (ICD-9-CM) codes: 070.41, 070.44, 070.51, 070.54, 070.70, 070.71, V02.62), were prescribed hepatoprotective agents (silymarin, liver hydrolysate, choline bitartrate, or ursodeoxycholic acid), but did not receive any anti-HCV therapy (ribavirin or peg-interferon). HCV-uninfected individuals were those who did not have a HCV diagnosis (ICD-9-CM) or tests for HCV infection, and received no hepatoprotective agents or anti-HCV therapy, and they were classified as being HCV-uninfected. The HCV-treated cohort was matched with untreated HCV-infected patients (HCV-untreated cohort) and with HCV-uninfected individuals (HCV-uninfected cohort) through a propensity score-matching method indicating the probability of receiving the combination therapy, estimated by using a logistic model. The covariates in the model included sex (male, female), age (20–39, 40–49, 50–59, $\geq$60), NHI registration location (city, township, rural area), Charlson Comorbidity Index (CCI) score (0, 1, $\geq$2), and year of the index date (2003–2006, 2007–2009, 2010–2012). This method was used to assure that the HCV-treated cohort and the selected counterparts were comparable in observed characteristics. The baselines for the HCV-untreated and HCV-uninfected cohorts were assigned according to the period from the index date to the baseline of their matched counterparts of the HCV-treated cohort, and subjects with rheumatic disease or mortality occurred before the baselines were not selected. The index date of the HCV-uninfected individuals was the date of one of their physician visits randomly selected from their claims database. The matching process for the 3 cohorts is shown in Supplementary Figure S1.

Outcomes were defined as the development of rheumatic diseases as mentioned above. Subjects were followed until the date of the event, death, or the end of follow-up (31 December 2015), whichever came first. Dates of death were adopted from the Death Registry database. For the HCV-treated group, only the rheumatic disease or mortality occurred 6 months after the complement of anti-HCV therapy (the baseline) were recorded.

2.2. Statistical Analysis

All statistical analyses were performed using the Statistical Analysis System (SAS version 9.4, SAS Institute Inc., Cary, NC, USA) software. Continuous variables were analyzed using a Student's *t*-test or analysis of variance, as appropriate, and categorical variables were analyzed using a Chi-square test or Fisher's exact test, as appropriate. Cumulative incidences of outcomes were estimated and compared by using the modified Kaplan–Meier method and the Gray method, with death being a competing risk event. Sub-distribution hazards models for competing risks, an extension of Cox proportional hazards models taking competing mortality into consideration, were used to estimate adjusted hazard ratio of developing rheumatic diseases, adjusting for age, sex, NHI registration location, the CCI score, year of the index date, and comorbid liver cirrhosis, chronic obstructive pulmonary disease (COPD), end-stage renal disease (ESRD), DM, hypertension, dyslipidemia, cardiovascular events (including percutaneous coronary intervention, coronary artery bypass graft, myocardial infarction, heart failure, cardiogenic shock, and peripheral vascular disease), stroke, nonalcoholic fatty liver disease (NAFLD), alcoholic liver disease (ALD), and autoimmune liver disease. Statistical significance was defined at the 5% level.

2.3. Ethics Approval and Consent to Participate

The study protocol conformed to the ethical guidelines of the 1975 Declaration of Helsinki and was approved by the local Institutional Review Board. The need for consent was waived because the national-level data used in this study were de-identified by encrypting personal identification information.

3. Results

3.1. Baseline Characteristics

From a total of 19,298,735 individuals between 1 January 2003 and 31 December 2015, 11,223,475 patients without HBV infection and baseline rheumatic diseases were identified; 104,281 patients with HCV infection and 11,119,194 patients without HCV infection were eligible for the study. Of all, 3 cohorts including HCV-treated (n = 6919), HCV-untreated (n = 27,676) and HCV-uninfected (n = 27,676) cohorts were enrolled (Figure 1). The 3 cohorts were matched with the propensity scores (1:4:4), did not differ in demographic factors, residency, CCI score and index year, which were the covariates in the models to calculate propensity scores, although baseline comorbidities were not similar (Table 1). Compared with HCV-untreated cohorts, the HCV-treated cohort had higher rates of baseline cirrhosis, comparable rates of COPD, but lower rates of other comorbidities. Compared with the HCV-uninfected cohort, the HCV-treated cohort had higher rates of most comorbidities including cirrhosis, comparable rates of DM and cardiovascular events, but lower rates of dyslipidemia and stroke. Compared with the HCV-uninfected cohort, the HCV-untreated cohort had higher rates of all baseline comorbidities except stroke. To lineate the HCV-associated complications, we compared the baseline factors between the HCV-infected cohort, which was a combination of the HCV-treated and HCV-untreated cohorts, and HCV-uninfected cohort. The HCV-infected cohort had higher rates of all baseline comorbidities except indifferent rates of dyslipidemia and lower rates of stroke than the HCV-uninfected cohort (Supplementary Figure S2).

Table 1. Baseline characteristics of the 3 HCV cohorts of TNHIRD.

	(1)	(2)	(3)	p Values		
	Treated	Untreated	Uninfected	(1)–(2)	(1)–(3)	(2)–(3)
n	6919	27,676	27,676			
Gender, n, (%)						
Male	3832, (55.38)	15,328, (55.38)	15,328, (55.38)	1	1	1
Female	3087, (44.62)	12,348, (44.62)	12,348, (44.62)			
Age range (years), n, (%)						
20–39	1312, (18.96)	5247, (18.96)	5248, (18.96)	1	1	1
40–49	1811, (26.17)	7243, (26.17)	7244, (26.17)			
50–59	2443, (35.31)	9774, (35.32)	9772, (35.31)			
≥60	1353, (19.55)	5412, (19.55)	5412, (19.55)			
Area, n, (%)						
city	1482, (21.42)	5928, (21.42)	5928, (21.42)	1	1	1
township	2174, (31.42)	8696, (31.42)	8696, (31.42)			
rural area	3263, (47.16)	13,052, (47.16)	13,052, (47.16)			
CCI score, n, (%)						
0	3443, (49.76)	13,774, (49.77)	13,772, (49.76)	0.9999	1	0.9998
1	2138, (30.90)	8550, (30.89)	8552, (30.90)			
≥2	1338, (19.34)	5352, (19.34)	5352, (19.34)			
index_year, n, (%)						
2003–2006	3601, (52.05)	14,404, (52.05)	14,404, (52.05)	0.9997	1	0.9992
2007–2009	2274, (32.87)	9099, (32.88)	9096, (32.87)			
2010–2012	1044, (15.09)	4173, (15.08)	4176, (15.09)			
Baseline factor, n, (%)						
Liver cirrhosis	695, (10.04)	1685, (6.09)	9, (0.03)	<0.0001	<0.0001	<0.0001
COPD	775, (11.2)	3160, (11.42)	2548, (9.21)	0.6114	<0.0001	<0.0001
ESRD	47, (0.68)	722, (2.61)	81, (0.29)	<0.0001	<0.0001	<0.0001
DM	1320, (19.08)	6166, (22.28)	5004, (18.08)	<0.0001	0.0549	<0.0001
Hypertension	2011, (29.06)	9485, (34.27)	7422, (26.82)	<0.0001	0.0002	<0.0001
Dyslipidemia	815, (11.78)	5268, (19.03)	4815, (17.4)	<0.0001	<0.0001	<0.0001
Cardiovascular events	165, (2.38)	1059, (3.83)	685, (2.48)	<0.0001	0.6642	<0.0001

Table 1. Cont.

	(1) Treated	(2) Untreated	(3) Uninfected	p Values (1)–(2)	(1)–(3)	(2)–(3)
Stroke	227, (3.28)	1369, (4.95)	1407, (5.08)	<0.0001	<0.0001	0.4593
NAFLD	724 (10.46)	2425 (8.76)	188 (0.68)	<0.0001	<0.0001	<0.0001
ALD	105 (1.52)	653 (2.36)	20 (0.07)	<0.0001	<0.0001	<0.0001
Autoimmune liver disease	0	0	0			

TNHIRD: Taiwan National Health Insurance Research Database; HCV: hepatitis C virus; CCI: Charlson Comorbidity Index; COPD: Chronic obstructive pulmonary disease; ESRD: end-stage renal disease; DM: diabetes mellitus; NAFLD: nonalcoholic fatty liver disease; ALD: alcoholic liver disease.

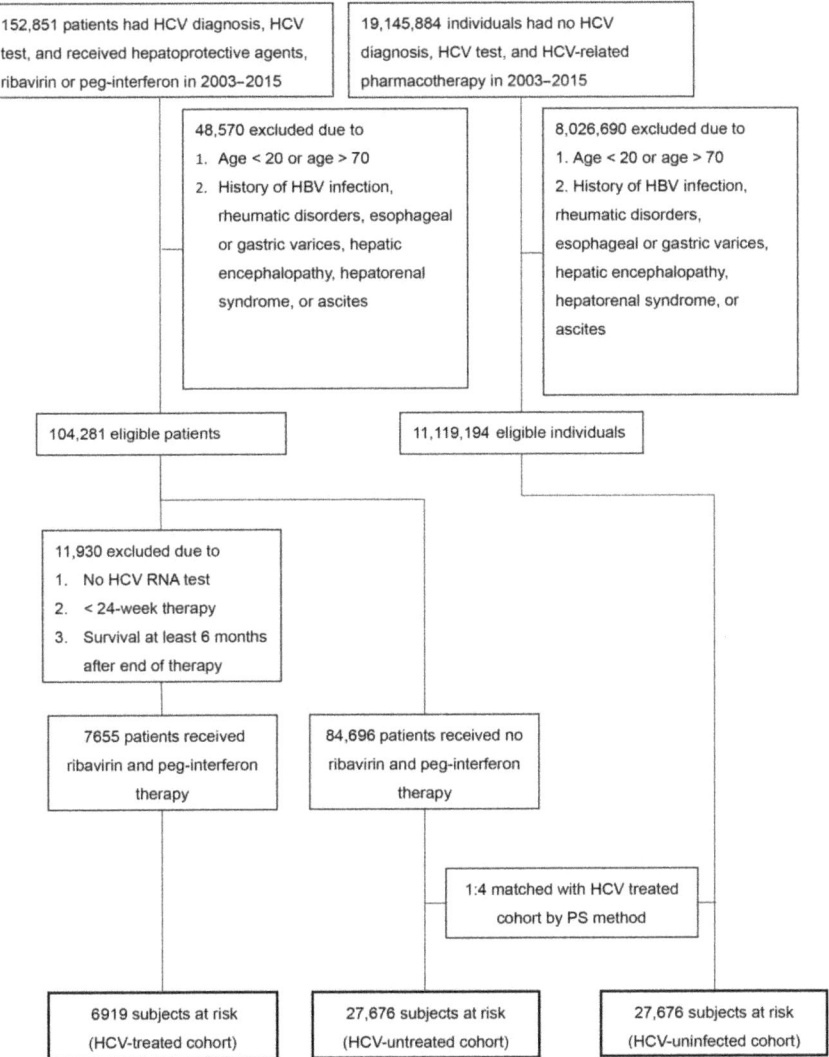

Figure 1. Flow chart of TNHIRD study subjects selection. TNHIRD: Taiwan National Health Insurance Research Database; HCV: hepatitis C virus; Peg-IFN: pegylated interferon; PS: propensity score.

3.2. Cumulative Incidences and Associated Factors of Rheumatic Diseases

The HCV-treated, -untreated, and -uninfected cohorts were followed up until 2015 or death, with the longest observation of 11 years. Rheumatic diseases occurred cumulatively at 11 years in 14.95%, 14.999%, and 9.535% of the HCV-treated, -untreated, and -uninfected cohorts, respectively (Figure 2, Table 2). The HCV-uninfected cohort had the lowest cumulative incidence of rheumatic diseases among the 3 cohorts. However, no difference of cumulative incidences of rheumatic diseases was identified between the HCV-treated and HCV-untreated cohorts. The multivariate analysis of the 3 cohorts showed, compared with the HCV-uninfected cohort, that both the HCV-treated and HCV-untreated cohorts had higher hazard ratios (HRs) to develop rheumatic disease. In addition, female sex, baseline age ≥ 49 years, CCI score ≥ 1, baseline COPD and dyslipidemia were associated with increased HRs of rheumatic diseases, while baseline liver cirrhosis, ESRD and DM were associated with decreased HRs of rheumatic diseases (Supplementary Figure S2). Given that HCV-treated and HCV-untreated cohorts yielded similar HRs to develop rheumatic diseases, we thus combined HCV-treated and HCV-untreated cohorts to form the HCV-infected cohort as mentioned above and compared the HCV-infected cohort with the HCV-uninfected cohort to view the impact of HCV infection on the development of rheumatic diseases. In addition to sex, age, CCI score, baseline COPD, dyslipidemia, cirrhosis, ESRD and DM, HCV infection was significantly associated with the development of rheumatic diseases, with a HR of 1.649 (Figure 3).

Table 2. Comparison of the cumulative incidences of rheumatic diseases among (1) HCV-treated, (2) HCV-untreated and (3) HCV-uninfected cohorts.

Rheumatic Disorders	(1) Treated	(2) Untreated	(3) Uninfected	*p* Values			
				(1)(2)(3)	(1)–(2)	(1)–(3)	(2)–(3)
Number	6919	27,676	27,676				
Follow-up (years), mean ± SD	4.61 ± 1.90	4.62 ± 1.07	4.89 ± 1.96				
Event number, *n* (%)	503 (7.27)	2140 (7.73)	1310 (4.73)				
Competing mortality, *n* (%)	281 (4.06)	3478 (12.57)	1316 (4.10)				
Cumulative incidence, % (95% CI)	14.95 (12.417–17.704)	14.999 (13.585–16.479)	9.535 (8.416–10.734)	<0.0001	0.8316	<0.0001	<0.0001

CI: confidence interval.

3.3. Cumulative Incidences of Mortality.

Of the 3 cohorts, the HCV-untreated cohort had the highest cumulative incidence (29.163%) of overall mortality at 11 years ($p < 0.0001$). The HCV-treated and HCV-uninfected cohorts yielded indifferent mortality rates ($p = 0.1796$) (Table 3).

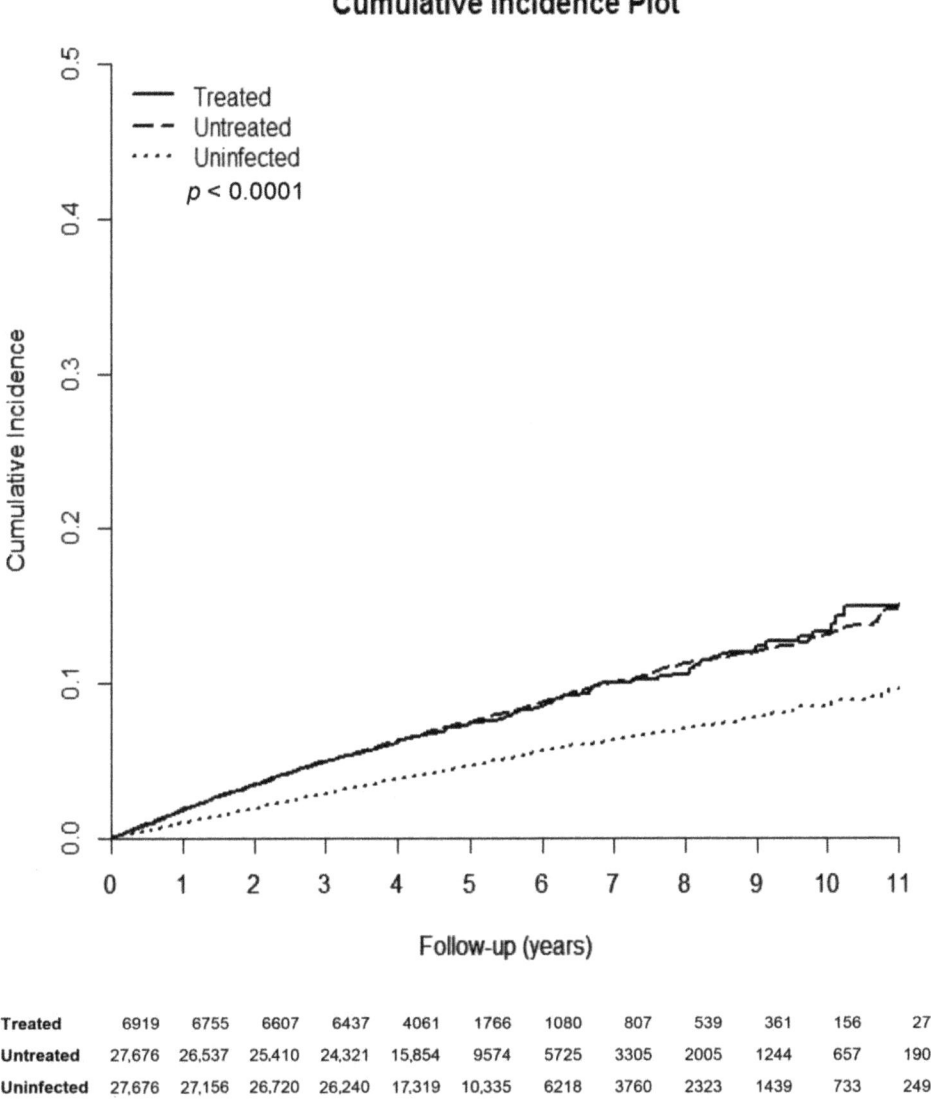

Figure 2. Cumulative incidences of rheumatic diseases among the 3 TNHIRD cohorts including HCV-treated, HCV-untreated and HCV-uninfected cohorts. TNHIRD: Taiwan National Health Insurance Research Database; HCV: hepatitis C virus.

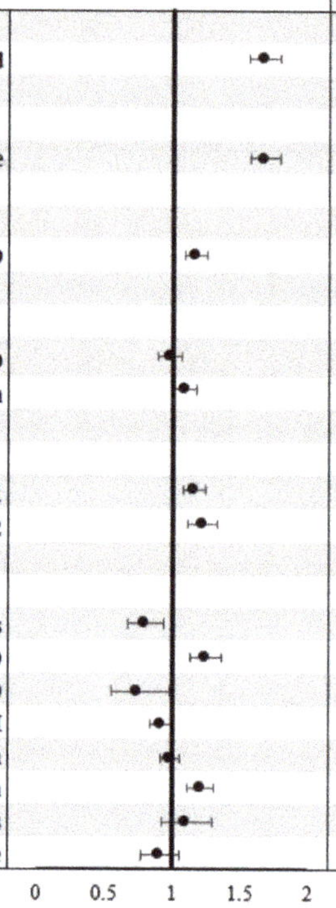

	HR	95% LCL	95% HCL	p value
HCV (ref = uninfected)				
infected	1.671	1.562	1.788	<0.0001
Gender (ref = Male)				
Female	1.670	1.565	1.782	<0.0001
Age (ref < 49)				
≥49	1.168	1.088	1.253	<0.0001
Area (ref = city)				
township	0.976	0.895	1.066	0.5924
rural area	1.082	0.997	1.173	0.0576
CCI score (ref = 0)				
1	1.156	1.074	1.245	0.0001
≥2	1.214	1.110	1.329	<0.0001
Baseline factor (ref = N)				
Liver cirrhosis	0.795	0.674	0.937	0.0062
COPD	1.244	1.134	1.364	<0.0001
ESRD	0.732	0.549	0.974	0.0326
DM	0.910	0.835	0.993	0.0333
Hypertension	0.979	0.908	1.055	0.5823
Dyslipidemia	1.205	1.108	1.310	<0.0001
Cardiovascular events	1.093	0.923	1.295	0.3033
Stroke	0.902	0.774	1.051	0.185

Figure 3. Forrest plot of factors associated with incident rheumatic diseases in the 2 TNHIRD cohorts: HCV-positive (untreated) and HCV-negative (combination of treated and uninfected) cohorts. TNHIRD: Taiwan National Health Insurance Research Database; HR: hazards ratio; LCL: lower confidence interval limit; HCL: higher confidence interval limit; HCV: hepatitis C virus; CCI: Charlson Comorbidity Index score; COPD: Chronic obstructive pulmonary disease; ESRD: end-stage renal disease; DM: diabetes mellitus; NAFLD: Nonalcoholic fatty liver disease; ALD: alcoholic liver disease.

Table 3. Comparison of the cumulative incidences of overall mortality among (1) HCV-treated, (2) HCV-untreated and (3) HCV-uninfected cohorts.

Overall Mortality	(1) Treated	(2) Untreated	(3) Uninfected	p Values			
				(1)(2)(3)	(1)–(2)	(1)–(3)	(2)–(3)
Number	6919	27,676	27,676				
Follow-up (years), mean ± SD	4.82 ± 1.84	4.86 ± 2.03	5.03 ± 1.91				
Event number, n (%)	304 (4.39)	3669 (13.26)	1170 (4.23)				
Cumulative incidence, % (95% CI)	13.662 (11.389–16.140)	29.163 (27.218–31.133)	9.99 (8.548–11.559)	<0.0001	<0.0001	0.1796	<0.0001

CI: confidence interval.

4. Discussion

The most compelling results of the current study are as follows: (1) The HCV-uninfected cohort had the lowest cumulative incidence of rheumatic diseases among the 3 cohorts, while indifferent cumulative incidences were identified between the HCV-treated and HCV-untreated cohorts. (2) HCV infection, female gender, baseline age ≥ 49 years, CCI score ≥ 1, baseline COPD and dyslipidemia were associated with increased HRs of rheumatic diseases, while baseline liver cirrhosis, ESRD and DM were associated with decreased HRs. (3) The HCV-untreated cohort had the highest cumulative incidence of overall mortality at 11 years, while HCV-treated and HCV-uninfected cohorts yielded indifferent mortality rates.

The higher rate of baseline cirrhosis in the HCV-treated than the HCV-untreated cohorts of TNHIRD was coincided with the fact that only patients with significant fibrosis were reimbursed with anti-HCV therapy [28], and the other different baseline variables between these 2 cohorts highlight the idea that patients with comorbidities were ineligible for the interferon-based therapy and had been excluded for anti-HCV therapy. The different rates in baseline variables between HCV-infected and HCV-uninfected cohorts were consistent with the phenomenon that HCV infection elicits many cardiometabolic events and hypolipidemia [1]. Therefore, the baseline comparisons of the 3 cohorts supported the reliability of the data based on TNHIRD.

The fact that the HCV-uninfected cohort had the lowest cumulative incidence of rheumatic diseases, and HCV infection increased the HR of developing rheumatic diseases based on multivariate analyses, endorsed the concept that HCV infection might cause rheumatic diseases, despite the fact that some studies did not support the participation of HCV infection in the pathogenesis of RA [29–31]. However, given that the HRs in developing rheumatic diseases between the HCV-treated and HCV-untreated cohorts were indifferent, the HCV-associated risk of rheumatic diseases might not be attenuated by interferon-based anti-HCV therapy. In particular, cryoglobulinemic vasculitis represents the prototype of HCV-related rheumatic diseases [3]; long-term mixed cryoglobulinemia after SVR is common since cryoglobulin-generating B lymphocytes might have reached an HCV-independent autonomous phase before viral clearance [32]. HCV-associated rheumatic disease therefore might persist despite viral clearance. Moreover, whether interferon-based therapy reduces the risk of RA had remained conflicting [33,34], and interferon-based anti-HCV therapy may work as a "trigger" for RA [35,36] or SLE [37] had been shown in some case reports. Although treatment with interferon-alpha may lead to substantial clinical improvement of HCV-related arthritis even without a complete biochemical or virological response [34], autoimmune diseases indeed occur in 4% to 19% of patients receiving interferon-based anti-HCV therapy and the associated symptoms developed between 2 weeks and 7 years after initiation of therapy [38].The interferon-based anti-HCV therapy thus has been contraindicated for many rheumatologic autoimmune/inflammatory diseases based on the concern of triggering rheumatic diseases. New oral interferon-free combinations of various DAAs offer an opportunity for HCV-infected patients with rheumatic diseases to be cured with a short treatment duration and a low risk of side effects [39]. However, SVR following DAA might lead to immune reconstitution as tuberculosis reactivation had been reported [40]. Whether DAA therapy precisely attenuates the risks of HCV-associated rheumatic disease without introducing other harm as mentioned above [40] demands further investigation.

On the other hand, that female sex and baseline age ≥ 49 years are positively associated with the increased HRs of rheumatic diseases is consistent with the fact that female sex and old age had been identified as risk factors for RA [41]. CCI score ≥ 1 and baseline COPD were associated with increased HRs of rheumatic diseases, which coincides with the fact that comorbidities including respiratory disease were more common in patients with RA at diagnosis than controls [42]. Patients with rheumatic diseases have increased prevalence of metabolic syndrome including dyslipidemia [43], and acute myocardial infarction risk increased by 38% [44] in RA patients might explain why dyslipidemia were associated with increased HR of rheumatic diseases. Of note, the fact that baseline liver cirrhosis, ESRD and DM are associated with reduced HRs of rheumatic diseases is a novel finding. Interestingly, the connections with cirrhosis are variable among different rheumatic diseases. For example, the overall incidences of cirrhosis were reported to be lower in the RA cohort than in the non-RA cohort [45,46], while patients with psoriasis were found to have increased risk of cirrhosis over patients without psoriasis [46].With regard to ESRD and DM, in contrast to their negative associations with the rheumatic disease risks, chronic kidney disease is a common complication of rheumatic diseases [47]; patients undergoing hemodialysis therapy may develop serious rheumatic complications [48], newly diagnosed RA patients are at higher risk of DM [49] and the prevalence of DM is higher in patients with psoriatic arthritis compared with the general population [50]. That rheumatic diseases might be mistaken as ESRD- or DM-related complications in patients with ESRD and DM potentially explains the aforementioned paradox.

Among the 3 cohorts, the HCV-untreated cohort yielded the highest overall mortality, which might be caused by other HCV-associated events such as cirrhosis, HCC or cardiometabolic events [1] other than rheumatic disease-associated complications, since HCV-treated and HCV-uninfected cohorts had indifferent mortalities, although the latter obviously had a lower risk of rheumatic diseases. This phenomenon indicates the importance to prescribe anti-HCV therapy in HCV-infected patients in decreasing overall mortality, regardless of the risk for rheumatic diseases.

There are limitations recognized in the current study. First, because linking the results from TNHIRD to the laboratory results of individual patients was forbidden for privacy protection, the correlation of SVR with rheumatic diseases could not be identified. However, we are confident in the antiviral efficacy in the HCV-treated cohort since interferon-based therapy for HCV infection generally achieves an SVR rate up to 90% in Taiwan [51], where a favorable genetic variation in IFNL3 is prevalent [51]. Second, as mentioned above, interferon-based therapy might elicit rheumatic diseases in SVR patients [35–38] and blunt the impact of viral clearance in attenuating rheumatic disease risks. Third, because most of the rheumatic diseases accounted for the minority of the whole population and our preliminary statistical tests did not show any significance for any individual rheumatic disease, we thus had put all rheumatic disorders together as rheumatic diseases to yield the maximal statistical power. Some specific rheumatic disorders might have different connections with HCV infection or anti-HCV therapy. Anyhow, that SVR did not reduce the incidences of SLE and RA in CHC patients [52] supported our observation. Future prospective studies in other independent large cohorts with identifiable SVR following DAA therapy, subgroup analyses for specific rheumatic disorders and sophisticated molecular investigations are required to elucidate the fundamental mechanisms underlying the findings described here.

Taken together, HCV infection, female sex, baseline age ≥ 49 years, and other comorbidities were associated with risks of rheumatic diseases. Although interferon-based therapy did not attenuate the rheumatic disease risk, it indeed decreased the overall mortality of HCV-infected patients. These findings may merit further study for preventing or treating rheumatic diseases in HCV-infected patients.

Supplementary Materials: The following are available online at https://www.mdpi.com/article/10.3390/jcm10040817/s1, Figure S1: Steps of the matching process, Figure S2: Comparison of the baseline factors between the HCV-infected cohort (HCV-treated and HCV-untreated cohorts), and HCV-uninfected cohort.

Author Contributions: Data curation, Y.-S.L., J.-H.H., M.-Y.C., H.-P.K., R.-N.C.; formal analysis, J.-S.C., H.-P.K., M.-L.C.; funding acquisition, M.-L.C.; investigation, M.-L.C.; methodology, M.-L.C.; supervision, M.-L.C. All authors have read and agreed to the published version of the manuscript.

Funding: This study was supported by grants from the Chang Gung Medical Research Program (CMRPG3I0412, CMRPG3K0721 and CMRPG1K0111) and the National Science Council (MOST 108-2314-B-182-051-, MOST 109-2314-B-182-024- and MOST 109-2629-B-182-002-). The funders had no role in study design, data collection and analysis, decision to publish, or preparation of the manuscript. The opinions expressed in this paper are those of the authors and do not necessarily represent those of the Chang Gung Medical Hospital and the National Science Council, Taiwan.

Institutional Review Board Statement: The study protocol conformed to the ethical guidelines of the 1975 Declaration of Helsinki and was approved by the local Institutional Review Board.

Informed Consent Statement: The need for consent was waived because the national-level data used in this study were de-identified by encrypting personal identification information.

Acknowledgments: The authors thank Shu-Chun Chen, Chia-Hui Tsai, Chun-Kai Liang and Shuen-Shian Shiau from the Liver Research Center, Chang Gung Memorial Hospital, Taiwan, for their assistance with data mining.

Conflicts of Interest: The authors declare no conflict of interest.

References

1. Chang, M.L. Metabolic alterations and hepatitis C: From bench to bedside. *World J. Gastroenterol.* **2016**, *22*, 1461–1476. [CrossRef]
2. Younossi, Z.M.; Henry, L.; Ong, P.J.; Tanaka, A.; Eguchi, Y.; Mizokami, M.; Lim, Y.-S.; Dan, Y.Y.; Yu, M.-L.; Stepanova, M. Systematic review with meta-analysis: Extrahepatic manifestations in chronic hepatitis C virus-infected patients in East Asia. *Aliment. Pharmacol. Ther.* **2019**, *49*, 644–653. [CrossRef]
3. Sebastiani, M.; Giuggioli, D.; Colaci, M.; Fallahi, P.; Gragnani, L.; Antonelli, A.; Zignego, A.L.; Ferri, C. HCV-related rheumatic manifestations and therapeutic strategies. *Curr. Drug Targets* **2017**, *18*, 803–810. [CrossRef]
4. Calvaruso, V.; Craxì, A. Immunological alterations in hepatitis C virus infection. *World J. Gastroenterol.* **2013**, *19*, 8916–8923. [CrossRef]
5. Sayiner, Z.A.; Haque, U.; Malik, M.U.; Gurakar, A. Hepatitis C virus infection and its rheumatologic implications. *Gastroenterol. Hepatol.* **2014**, *10*, 287–293.
6. Cacoub, P.; Renou, C.; Rosenthal, E.; Cohen, P.; Loury, I.; Loustaud-Ratti, V.; Yamamoto, A.-M.; Camproux, A.-C.; Hausfater, P.; Musset, L.; et al. Extrahepatic manifestations associated with hepatitis C virus infection. A prospective multicenter study of 321 patients. *Medicine* **2000**, *79*, 47–56. [CrossRef]
7. Mohammed, R.H.; ElMakhzangy, H.I.; Gamal, A.; Mekky, F.; El Kassas, M.; Mohammed, N.; Hamid, A.M.; Esmat, G. Prevalence of rheumatologic manifestations of chronic hepatitis C virus infection among Egyptians. *Clin.Rheumatol.* **2010**, *29*, 1373–1380. [CrossRef]
8. Palazzi, C.; Olivieri, I.; Cacciatore, P.; Pennese, E.; D'Amico, E. Difficulties in the differential diagnosis between primitive rheumatic diseases and hepatitis C virus-related disorders. *Clin. ExpRheumatol.* **2005**, *23*, 2–6.
9. El Garf, A.; El Zorkany, B.; Gheith, R.; Sheba, H.; Abdel Moneim, G.; El Garf, K. Prevalence and clinical presentations of hepatitis C virus among patients admitted to the rheumatology ward. *Rheumatol. Int.* **2012**, *32*, 2691–2695. [CrossRef] [PubMed]
10. MohdHanafiah, K.; Groeger, J.; Flaxman, A.D.; Wiersma, S.T. Global epidemiology of hepatitis C virus infection: New estimates of age-specific antibody to HCV seroprevalence. *Hepatology* **2013**, *57*, 1333–1342. [CrossRef] [PubMed]
11. Ramos-Casals, M.; Muñoz, S.; Medina, F.; Jara, L.-J.; Rosas, J.; Calvo-Alen, J.; Brito-Zerón, P.; Forns, X.; Sánchez-Tapias, J.-M. Systemic autoimmune diseases in patients with hepatitis C virus infection: Characterization of 1020 cases (The HISPAMEC Registry). *J. Rheumatol.* **2009**, *36*, 1442–1448. [CrossRef] [PubMed]
12. Pawlotsky, J.M.; Ben Yahia, M.; Andre, C.; Voisin, M.C.; Intrator, L.; Roudot-Thoraval, F.; Deforges, L.; Duvoux, C.; Zafrani, E.-S.; Duval, J.; et al. Immunological disorders in C virus chronic active hepatitis: A prospective case-control study. *Hepatology* **1994**, *19*, 841–848. [CrossRef] [PubMed]
13. Loustaud-Ratti, V.; Riche, A.; Liozon, E.; Labrousse, F.; Soria, P.; Rogez, S.; Babany, G.; Delaire, L.; Denis, F.; Vidal, E. Prevalence and characteristics of Sjögren's syndrome or Sicca syndrome in chronic hepatitis C virus infection: A prospective study. *J. Rheumatol.* **2001**, *28*, 2245–2251. [PubMed]
14. Brito-Zerón, P.; Gheitasi, H.; Retamozo, S.; Bové, A.; Londoño, M.; Sánchez-Tapias, J.-M.; Caballero, M.; Kostov, B.; Forns, X.; Kaveri, S.V.; et al. How hepatitis C virus modifies the immunological profile of Sjögrensyndrome: Analysis of 783 patients. *Arthritis Res.Ther.* **2015**, *17*, 250. [CrossRef]
15. Cacoub, P.; Poynard, T.; Ghillani, P.; Charlotte, F.; Olivi, M.; Piette, J.C.; Opolon, P. Extrahepatic manifestations of chronic hepatitis C. *Arthritis Rheum.* **1999**, *42*, 2204–2212. [CrossRef]
16. Su, F.H.; Wu, C.S.; Sung, F.C.; Chang, S.N.; Su, C.T.; Shieh, Y.H.; Yeh, C.-C. Chronic hepatitis C virus infection is associated with the development of rheumatoid arthritis: A nationwide population-based study in taiwan. *PLoS ONE* **2014**, *9*, e113579. [CrossRef]
17. Kudaeva, F.M.; Speechley, M.R.; Pope, J.E. A systematic review of viral exposures as a risk for rheumatoid arthritis. *Semin. Arthritis Rheum.* **2019**, *48*, 587–596. [CrossRef] [PubMed]
18. Mercado, U.; Avendaño-Reyes, M.; Araiza-Casillas, R.; Díaz-Molina, R. Prevalance of antibodies against hepatitis C and B viruses in patients with systemic lupus erythematosus. *Rev. Gastroenterol. Mex.* **2005**, *70*, 399–401. (In Spanish)
19. Vermehren, J.; Park, J.S.; Jacobson, I.M.; Zeuzem, S. Challenges and perspectives of direct antivirals for the treatment of hepatitis C virus infection. *J. Hepatol.* **2018**, *69*, 1178–1187. [CrossRef]
20. Toyoda, H.; Kumada, T.; Tada, T.; Kiriyama, S.; Tanikawa, M.; Hisanaga, Y.; Kanamori, A.; Kitabatake, S.; Ito, T. Risk factors of hepatocellular carcinoma development in non-cirrhotic patients with sustained virologic response for chronic hepatitis C virus infection. *J. Gastroenterol. Hepatol.* **2015**, *30*, 1183–1189. [CrossRef]
21. Kalaitzakis, E.; Gunnarsdottir, S.A.; Josefsson, A.; Björnsson, E. Increased risk for malignant neoplasms among patients with cirrhosis. *Clin. Gastroenterol. Hepatol.* **2011**, *9*, 168–174. [CrossRef]
22. Hu, J.H.; Chen, M.Y.; Yeh, C.T.; Lin, H.S.; Lin, M.S.; Huang, T.J.; Chang, M.-L. Sexual dimorphic metabolic alterations in hepatitis C virus-infected patients: A community-based study in a hepatitis B/hepatitis C virus hyperendemic area. *Medicine* **2016**, *95*, e3546. [CrossRef] [PubMed]

23. Chang, M.-L.; Lin, Y.-J.; Chang, C.-J.; Yeh, C.; Chen, T.-C.; Yeh, T.-S.; Lee, W.-C.; Yeh, C.-T. Occult and overt HBV co-infections independently predict postoperative prognosis in HCV-associated hepatocellular carcinoma. *PLoS ONE* **2013**, *8*, e64891. [CrossRef]
24. Mathieu, A.; Paladini, F.; Vacca, A.; Cauli, A.; Fiorillo, M.T.; Sorrentino, R. The interplay between the geographic distribution of HLA-B27 alleles and their role in infectious and autoimmune diseases: A unifying hypothesis. *Autoimmun. Rev.* **2009**, *8*, 420–425. [CrossRef] [PubMed]
25. Aksu, K.; Kabasakal, Y.; Sayiner, A.; Keser, G.; Oksel, F.; Bilgiç, A.; Gümüşdiş, G.; Doganavşargil, E. Prevalences of hepatitis A, B, C and E viruses in Behçet's disease. *Rheumatology* **1999**, *38*, 1279–1281. [CrossRef] [PubMed]
26. Ferri, C.; Sebastiani, M.; Antonelli, A.; Colaci, M.; Manfredi, A.; Giuggioli, D. Current treatment of hepatitis C-associated rheumatic diseases. *Arthritis Res. Ther.* **2012**, *14*, 215. [CrossRef]
27. Noe, M.H.; Grewal, S.K.; Shin, D.B.; Ogdie, A.; Takeshita, J.; Gelfand, J.M. Increased prevalence of HCV and hepatic decompensation in adults with psoriasis: A population-based study in the United Kingdom. *J. Eur. Acad. Dermatol. Venereol.* **2017**, *31*, 1674–1680. [CrossRef]
28. Chen, C.W.; Cheng, J.S.; Chen, T.D.; Le, P.H.; Ku, H.P.; Chang, M.L. The irreversible HCV-associated risk of gastric cancer following interferon-based therapy: A joint study of hospital-based cases and nationwide population-based cohorts. *Therap. Adv. Gastroenterol.* **2019**, *12*, 1756284819855732. [CrossRef]
29. Yılmaz, N.; Karadağ, Ö.; Kimyon, G.; Yazıcı, A.; Yılmaz, S.; Kalyoncu, U.; Kaşifoğlu, T.; Temiz, H.; Baysal, B.; Tözün, N. Prevalence of hepatitis B and C infections in rheumatoid arthritis and ankylosing spondylitis: A multicenter countrywide study. *Eur. J. Rheumatol.* **2014**, *1*, 51–54. [CrossRef]
30. Maillefert, J.F.; Muller, G.; Falgarone, G.; Bour, J.B.; Ratovohery, D.; Dougados, M.; Tavernier, C.; Breban, M. Prevalence of hepatitis C virus infection in patients with rheumatoid arthritis. *Ann. Rheum. Dis.* **2002**, *61*, 635–637. [CrossRef]
31. Hsu, F.C.; Starkebaum, G.; Boyko, E.J.; Dominitz, J.A. Prevalence of rheumatoid arthritis and hepatitis C in those age 60 and older in a US population based study. *J.Rheumatol.* **2003**, *30*, 455–458.
32. Cheng, Y.T.; Cheng, J.S.; Lin, C.H.; Chen, T.H.; Lee, K.C.; Chang, M.L. Rheumatoid factor and immunoglobulin M mark hepatitis C-associated mixed cryoglobulinaemia: An 8-year prospective study. *Clin. Microbiol. Infect.* **2020**, *26*, 366–372. [CrossRef] [PubMed]
33. Tung, C.H.; Lai, N.S.; Li, C.Y.; Tsai, S.J.; Chen, Y.C.; Chen, Y.C. Risk of rheumatoid arthritis in patients with hepatitis C virus infection receiving interferon-based therapy: A retrospective cohort study using the Taiwanese national claims database. *BMJ Open* **2018**, *8*, e021747. [CrossRef]
34. Rossi, C.; Jeong, D.; Wong, S.; McKee, G.; Butt, Z.A.; Buxton, J.; Wong, J.; Darvishian, M.; Bartlett, S.; Samji, H.; et al. Sustained virological response from interferon-based hepatitis C regimens is associated with reduced risk of extrahepatic manifestations. *J. Hepatol.* **2019**, *71*, 1116–1125. [CrossRef]
35. Izumi, Y.; Komori, A.; Yasunaga, Y.; Hashimoto, S.; Miyashita, T.; Abiru, S.; Yatsuhashi, H.; Ishibashi, H.; Migita, K. Rheumatoid arthritis following a treatment with IFN-alpha/ribavirin against HCV infection. *Intern Med.* **2011**, *50*, 1065–1068. [CrossRef]
36. Pittau, E.; Bogliolo, A.; Tinti, A.; Mela, Q.; Ibba, G.; Salis, G.; Perpignano, G. Development of arthritis and hypothyroidism during alpha-interferon therapy for chronic hepatitis C. *Clin. Exp. Rheumatol.* **1997**, *15*, 415–419.
37. Niewold, T.B.; Swedler, W.I. Systemic lupus erythematosus arising during interferon-alpha therapy for cryoglobulinemic vasculitis associated with hepatitis C. *Clin. Rheumatol.* **2005**, *24*, 178–181. [CrossRef]
38. Wilson, L.E.; Widman, D.; Dikman, S.H.; Gorevic, P.D. Autoimmune disease complicating antiviral therapy for hepatitis C virus infection. *Semin. Arthritis Rheum.* **2002**, *32*, 163–173. [CrossRef]
39. Cacoub, P.; Comarmond, C.; Desbois, A.C.; Saadoun, D. Rheumatologic manifestations of hepatitis C virus infection. *Clin. Liver Dis.* **2017**, *21*, 455–464. [CrossRef] [PubMed]
40. Kida, T.; Umemura, A.; Kaneshita, S.; Sagawa, R.; Inoue, T.; Toyama, S.; Wada, M.; Kohno, M.; Oda, R.; Inaba, T.; et al. Effectiveness and safety of chronic hepatitis C treatment with direct-acting antivirals in patients with rheumatic diseases: A case-series. *Mod. Rheumatol.* **2020**, *30*, 1009–1015. [CrossRef] [PubMed]
41. Safiri, S.; Kolahi, A.A.; Hoy, D.; Smith, E.; Bettampadi, D.; Mansournia, M.A.; Almasi-Hashiani, A.; Ashrafi-Asgarabad, A.; Moradi-Lakeh, M.; Qorbani, M.; et al. Global, regional and national burden of rheumatoid arthritis 1990–2017: A systematic analysis of the Global Burden of Disease study 2017. *Ann. Rheum. Dis.* **2019**, *78*, 1463–1471. [CrossRef]
42. Nikiphorou, E.; De Lusignan, S.; Mallen, C.; Roberts, J.; Khavandi, K.; Bedarida, G.; Buckley, C.D.; Galloway, J.; Raza, K. Prognostic value of comorbidity indices and lung diseases in early rheumatoid arthritis: A UK population-based study. *Rheumatology* **2020**, *59*, 1296–1305. [CrossRef]
43. Medina, G.; Vera-Lastra, O.; Peralta-Amaro, A.L.; Jiménez-Arellano, M.P.; Saavedra, M.A.; Cruz-Domínguez, M.P.; Jara, L.J. Metabolic syndrome, autoimmunity and rheumatic diseases. *Pharmacol. Res.* **2018**, *133*, 277–288. [CrossRef] [PubMed]
44. Chung, W.-S.; Lin, C.-L.; Peng, C.-L.; Chen, Y.-F.; Lu, C.-C.; Sung, F.-C.; Kao, C.-H. Rheumatoid arthritis and risk of acute myocardial infarction—A nationwide retrospective cohort study. *Int. J. Cardiol.* **2013**, *168*, 4750–4754. [CrossRef] [PubMed]
45. Hsu, C.S.; Lang, H.C.; Huang, K.Y.; Chao, Y.C.; Chen, C.L. Risks of hepatocellular carcinoma and cirrhosis-associated complications in patients with rheumatoid arthritis: A 10-year population-based cohort study in Taiwan. *Hepatol. Int.* **2018**, *12*, 531–543. [CrossRef]
46. Tung, C.H.; Lai, N.S.; Lu, M.C.; Lee, C.C. Liver cirrhosis in selected autoimmune diseases: A nationwide cohort study in Taiwan. *Rheumatol. Int.* **2016**, *36*, 199–205. [CrossRef] [PubMed]

47. Ciszek, M.; Kisiel, B.; Czerwinski, J.; Hryniewiecka, E.; Lewandowska, D.; Borczon, S.; Tlustochowicz, W.; Pączek, L. Kidney transplant recipients with rheumatic diseases: Epidemiological data from the Polish transplant registries 1998–2015. *Transpl. Proc.* **2018**, *50*, 1654–1657. [CrossRef] [PubMed]
48. Akasbi, N.; Houssaini, T.S.; Tahiri, L.; Hachimi, H.; El Maaroufi, C.; El Youbi, R.; Arrayhani, M.; Harzy, T. Rheumatic complications of long term treatment with hemodialysis. *Rheumatol. Int.* **2012**, *32*, 1161–1163. [CrossRef] [PubMed]
49. Emamifar, A.; Levin, K.; Jensen Hansen, I.M. Patients with newly diagnosed rheumatoid arthritis are at increased risk of diabetes mellitus: An observational cohort study. *Acta Reumatol. Port.* **2017**, *42*, 310–317. [PubMed]
50. Eder, L.; Chandran, V.; Cook, R.; Gladman, D.D. The risk of developing diabetes mellitus in patients with psoriatic arthritis: A cohort study. *J. Rheumatol.* **2017**, *44*, 286–291. [CrossRef]
51. Yu, M.-L.; Dai, C.-Y.; Huang, J.-F.; Hou, N.-J.; Lee, L.-P.; Hsieh, M.-Y.; Chiu, C.-F.; Lin, Z.-Y.; Chen, S.-C.; Wang, L.-Y.; et al. A randomised study of peginterferon and ribavirin for 16 versus 24 weeks in patients with genotype 2 chronic hepatitis C. *Gut* **2007**, *56*, 553–559. [CrossRef] [PubMed]
52. Hsu, W.-F.; Chen, C.-Y.; Tseng, K.-C.; Lai, H.-C.; Kuo, H.-T.; Hung, C.-H.; Tung, S.-Y.; Wang, J.-H.; Chen, J.-J.; Lee, P.-L.; et al. Sustained virological response to hepatitis C therapy does not decrease the incidence of systemic lupus erythematosus or rheumatoid arthritis. *Sci. Rep.* **2020**, *10*, 5372. [CrossRef] [PubMed]

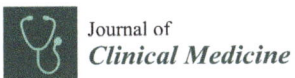

Article

Phylogenetic and Molecular Analyses of More Prevalent HCV1b Subtype in the Calabria Region, Southern Italy

Nadia Marascio [1,*,†], Angela Costantino [2,†], Stefania Taffon [2], Alessandra Lo Presti [2], Michele Equestre [3], Roberto Bruni [2], Giulio Pisani [4], Giorgio Settimo Barreca [1], Angela Quirino [1], Enrico Maria Trecarichi [5], Chiara Costa [5], Maria Mazzitelli [5], Francesca Serapide [5], Giovanni Matera [1], Carlo Torti [5], Maria Carla Liberto [1] and Anna Rita Ciccaglione [2]

1. Department of Health Sciences, Institute of Microbiology, "Magna Grecia" University, 88100 Catanzaro, Italy; gbarreca@unicz.it (G.S.B.); quirino@unicz.it (A.Q.); gm4106@gmail.com (G.M.); mliberto@unicz.it (M.C.L.)
2. Department of Infectious Diseases, Istituto Superiore di Sanità, 00161 Rome, Italy; angela.costantino@iss.it (A.C.); stefania.taffon@iss.it (S.T.); alessandra.lopresti@iss.it (A.L.P.); roberto.bruni@iss.it (R.B.); annarita.ciccaglione@iss.it (A.R.C.)
3. Department of Cell Biology and Neuroscience, Istituto Superiore di Sanità, 00161 Rome, Italy; michele.equestre@iss.it
4. National Center for Immunobiologicals Research and Evaluation, Istituto Superiore di Sanità, 00161 Rome, Italy; giulio.pisani@iss.it
5. Department of Medical and Surgical Sciences, Unit of Infectious and Tropical Diseases, "Magna Graecia" University, 88100 Catanzaro, Italy; em.trecarichi@unicz.it (E.M.T.); c.costa@materdominiaou.it (C.C.); m.mazzitelli88@gmail.com (M.M.); francescaserapide@gmail.com (F.S.); torti@unicz.it (C.T.)
* Correspondence: nmarascio@unicz.it; Tel.: +39-0961-3697-742; Fax: +39-0961-3697-760
† Contributed equally.

Abstract: Hepatitis C virus subtype 1b (HCV1b) is still the most prevalent subtype worldwide, with massive expansion due to poor health care standards, such as blood transfusion and iatrogenic procedures. Despite safe and effective new direct antiviral agents (DAA), treatment success can depend on resistance-associated substitutions (RASs) carried in target genomic regions. Herein we investigated transmission clusters and RASs among isolates from HCV1b positive subjects in the Calabria Region. Forty-one NS5B and twenty-two NS5A sequences were obtained by Sanger sequencing. Phylogenetic analysis was performed using the maximum likelihood method and resistance substitutions were analyzed with the Geno2pheno tool. Phylogenetic analysis showed sixteen statistically supported clusters, with twelve containing Italian sequences mixed with foreign HCV1b isolates and four monophyletic clusters including only sequences from Calabria. Interestingly, HCV1b spread has been maintained by sporadic infections in geographically limited areas and by dental treatment or surgical intervention in the metropolitan area. The L159F NS5B RAS was found in 15 isolates and in particular 8/15 also showed the C316N substitution. The Y93H and L31M NS5A RASs were detected in three and one isolates, respectively. The A92T NS5A RAS was found in one isolate. Overall, frequencies of detected NS5B and NS5A RASs were 36.6% and 22.7%, respectively. For the eradication of infection, improved screening policies should be considered and the prevalence of natural RASs carried on viral strains.

Keywords: hepatitis C virus (HCV); phylogeny; resistance-associated substitution (RAS)

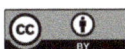

1. Introduction

Hepatitis C (HCV) infection remains a major public health problem, even if in the last few years HCV therapy has been improved by the availability of direct-acting antiviral (DAA) agents [1]. Phylogenetic analyses have identified eight HCV major genotypes, further subdivided into 67 subtypes [2]. HCV1b is widespread all over the world, HCV2 showed higher prevalence in Russia and in Italy. In Europe, the most common HCV2 subtypes are HCV2a/2c. HCV1a and HCV3a predominate in Europe and North America, while HCV4 is endemic in the Middle East, Central Africa and Mediterranean countries. HCV5 is endemic in South Africa, HCV6 in South East Asia and HCV7 was found in the Democratic Republic of Congo. Recently, HCV8 was found in Indian patients living in Canada [2–4]. Magiorkinis and colleagues reported a massive expansion of HCV1b infections between 1940 and 1980, sustained by blood transfusion and iatrogenic procedures [5]. In Europe, HCV1b was predominantly found in females and associated with births not later than 1958 [4]. Its prevalence is decreasing due to improved health standards [6]. Interestingly, HCV1b was predominant in Japan, Italy, and Spain with a high prevalence in patients with hepatocellular carcinoma [7]. Since 1997, HCV1b has been the most prevalent subtype in the Calabria Region reflecting national data [3,8].

The major prevalence worldwide and the low susceptibility to Interferon (IFN) or pegylated-IFN alfa with ribavirin (pegIFN-α/RBV) therapies made HCV1b the first target for the development of new antiviral drugs [9]. Currently, direct-acting-antiviral (DAA) pan-genotypic therapy can be used to treat infected people without the need for determining the genotype/subtype or performing a resistance test [1]. Pretreatment assessment should consider the presence of cirrhosis and comorbidity in view of post-therapy follow-up. However, after considering the data of DAA efficacy in a clinical setting, combination therapy still appears to be influenced by resistance-associated substitutions (RASs) carried in target regions in naïve or experienced patients [10].

In this study, we investigated transmission clusters in two cohorts of HCV1b positive subjects, enrolled in different time spans, to assess the dynamics of infection in the Calabria Region, southern Italy. In particular, more recent isolates were evaluated for the presence of mutations with a potential impact on treatment response.

2. Materials and Methods

2.1. Study Population

The study was approved by the Ethical Committee (#100; 27 April 2017) of the "Mater Domini" University Teaching Hospital of Catanzaro, Italy and it was included in the SINERGIE study [11]. The Ethical Committee approved the criteria that there is no need for informed consent for a non-interventional study. Forty-one serum samples, collected between 1 January 2015 and 31 December 2016, from patients infected by HCV subtype 1b were included in the analysis. Enrolled patients, attending the University Hospital of Catanzaro, were randomly selected from a list through a systematic 1:7 sampling procedure. The selected sample is representative of the whole HCV1b cohort, including 41.7% of males versus 54.0% of females with an overall median age 68 (31–84) years [12]. Patients were naïve to all treatments (25/41) or treated with IFN (3/41) and pegIFN-α/RBV (13/41). Additionally, only viral isolates from HCV1b positive subjects, collected between May and October 2010 during a previous epidemiological study in Calabria, were included in order to compare and investigate phylogenetic relationships with those from Catanzaro. All participants were resident in a small village, Sersale (Catanzaro province) [13]. The patients' clinical data was treated in accordance with the Helsinki Declaration (59th World Medical Association General Assembly, Seoul, Korea, October 2008) and the principles of good clinical practice.

2.2. Diagnostic Procedures

HCV RNA viral load was determined using the Cobas AmpliPrep/Cobas TaqMan HCV quantitative test v2.0 (Roche Diagnostics, Milan, Italy). Genotyping was performed by the Versant HCV genotype v2.0 assay (LiPA) (Siemens, Healthcare Diagnostic Inc., Tarrytown, NY, USA). Fibrosis stage was estimated by transient elastometry (FibroScan, Echosens, Paris, France), interpreted as follows: F0–F1 = minimal fibrosis (KPa $\leq$ 7.1), F2 = moderate fibrosis (7.1 < KPa $\leq$ 9.5), F3 = severe fibrosis (9.5 < KPa $\leq$ 14.5), F4 = cirrhosis (KPa > 14.5) [14].

2.3. Amplification and Sequencing of HCV NS5B and NS5A Regions

Viral RNA was extracted from 140 µL serum samples using the QIAamp Viral RNA Extraction Kit (Qiagen, Hilden, Germany) in accordance with the manufacturer's instructions. Healthy donor serum samples were used as a negative control. The RNA was reverse transcribed using the High-Capacity cDNA Reverse Transcription Kit protocol (Thermo Fischer Scientific, Waltham, MA, USA) and cDNA amplified by nested PCR using the FastStart High Fidelity PCR system (Roche Diagnostics, Basel, Switzerland). The specific primers used to amplify the NS5B (nt 8256–8632) and NS5A (nt 6086–6722) regions of HCV genome for the first and second rounds have been previously described [15,16]. The products were purified using the High Pure PCR Cleanup Micro Kit (Roche Diagnostics, Basel, Switzerland) and analyzed on 2% agarose gel stained with GelRed (Biotium Corporete Headquarters, Biotium Inc., Fremont, CA, USA). Both strands were sequenced using the Genome Lab DTCS Quick Start KiT (Beckman Coulter, Inc., Fullerton, CA, USA). Sequencing reactions were run on an automated DNA sequencer (Beckman Coulter, Inc., Fullerton, CA, USA). HCV sequences were aligned by MAFFT under the Galaxy platform (https://usegalaxy.org/, accessed on 27 March 2020) and manually edited by using Bioedit [17–19].

2.4. Subtyping Tool Analysis

NS5B and NS5A sequences were analyzed using the Oxford HCV Automated Subtyping Tool v.2.0 (http://dbpartners.stanford.edu/RegaSubtyping/html/subtypinghcvSUB.html, accessed on 20 April 2020) and COMET HCV typing tool (https://comet.lih.lu/index.php?cat=hcv, accessed on 20 April 2020) followed by phylogenetic analysis (see below) to confirm the initial subtyping assignment by LiPA assay [20,21].

2.5. Datasets Construction

Two datasets were built. The first dataset contained 78 total sequences: 53 HCV NS5B new sequences from Italy (41 from Catanzaro University Hospital and 12 from Sersale) plus 25 HCV NS5B subtype specific reference sequences downloaded from the HCV Los Alamos sequence database (http://hcv.lanl.gov/content/index, accessed on 11 May 2020). The second dataset comprised 162 total sequences including: 53 HCV NS5B sequences from Italy, previously classified as 1b subtype, plus 109 foreign HCV 1b NS5B sequences downloaded from the HCV Los Alamos sequence database (http://hcv.lanl.gov/content/index, accessed on 11 May 2020).

2.6. Likelihood Mapping

The phylogenetic signal of each sequence dataset was investigated by means of the likelihood mapping analysis of 10,000 random quartets generated using TreePuzzle [22]. Groups of four randomly chosen sequences (quartets) were evaluated. For each quartet, the three possible unrooted trees were reconstructed using the maximum likelihood approach under the selected substitution model. Posterior probabilities of each tree were then plotted on a triangular surface so that fully resolved trees fell into the corners and the unresolved quartets in the center of the triangle (star-like trees). When using this strategy, if more than 30% of the dots fall into the center of the triangle, the data is considered unreliable for the purposes of phylogenetic inference.

2.7. Phylogenetic Analysis

Sequences of all datasets were aligned using MAFFT under the Galaxy platform and manually edited using Bioedit [17–19]. The subtypes of the newly generated sequences from Calabria were determined and confirmed by phylogenetic analysis of the first dataset. The maximum likelihood phylogenetic trees of the first and second dataset together with the estimation of the best-fit substitution models (TPM2 + F + I + G4 and TVMe + I + G4 for the first and second dataset, respectively) were performed through IQ-TREE with the Model Finder option and visualized with FigTree v. 1.4.4 [23]. Statistical support for internal branches of the maximum likelihood (ML) trees were evaluated by bootstrap analysis (1000 replicates) and fast likelihood-based sh-like probability (SH-aLRT).

2.8. Genetic Variability Analysis

HCV1b viral population for each patient was screened for genetic variation with a cut-off of 15% [1]. Forty-one NS5B and twenty-two NS5A sequences at specific nucleotide positions were analyzed. Non-synonymous and resistance-associated substitutions (RAS) were determined using the Geno2pheno (HCV) 0.92 tool (last updated: June 2019) and aligning generated sequences to HCV1b (AJ238799) reference by MAFFT [17,24]. Resistance prediction rules available in the online tool were implemented by literature search [25].

2.9. Public Availability of the Sequencing Data

The 41 NS5B and 22 NS5A newly generated sequences were submitted to the GenBank database [26]. All sequences can be retrieved from GenBank under accession numbers: MW357752-MW357814.

3. Results

3.1. Patient Demographic Characteristics and Risk Factors

The median age of the 53 patients was 70 years (range 31–90), with 58.5% females. Overall, dental treatment and surgical intervention were the first (16.9%) and second (13.2%) most frequent risk factors, followed by blood transfusion (3.8%) and cohabitation (1.9%). Only one patient reported intravenous drug use as a risk factor. Three patients declared no risk factors. Qualitative characteristics of the two cohorts are reported separately (Table 1).

Table 1. Patient demographic characteristics.

	Absolute Number (%)		
Characteristics	Overall	Patients from University Hospital	Subjects from Sersale Village
Gender			
M	22 (41.5)	21 (48.7)	1 (8.3)
F	31 (58.5)	20 (51.3)	11 (91.7)
Risk factors			
Surgical intervention	7 (13.2)	7 (17.1)	-
Blood transfusion	2 (3.8)	2 (4.8)	-
Dental treatment therapy	9 (16.9)	9 (21.9)	-
Cohabitation	1 (1.9)	1 (2.4)	-
Multiple *	31 (58.5)	22 (53.6)	9 (75)
Not available	3 (5.7)	-	3 (25)
Clinical parameters			
cirrhotic status	-	14 (34.1)	not available
HCV RNA median level	3,792,576 IU/mL	2,280,000 IU/mL	3,918,625 IU/mL
Median (range)			
Age (years)	70 (31–90)	68 (31–85)	71 (65–90)
Total	53	41	12

* Multiple risk factors were: surgical intervention + blood transfusion (*n* = 4), surgical intervention + blood transfusion + cohabitation (*n* = 2), blood transfusion + cohabitation (*n* = 1), blood transfusion + dental treatment (*n* = 2), dental treatment + cohabitation (*n* = 1), surgical intervention + cohabitation (*n* = 2), surgical intervention + dental treatment (*n* = 8), surgical intervention + drug user (*n* = 1), surgical intervention + dental treatment + cohabitation (*n* = 1), surgical intervention + glass syringes (*n* = 7), surgical intervention + cohabitation + blood transfusion + glass syringes (*n* = 1), cohabitation + glass syringes (*n* = 1). Characteristics heading and total number of patients were in bold.

3.2. Likelihood Mapping

The phylogenetic noise of each dataset was investigated by means of likelihood mapping (Figure S1). The percentage of dots falling in the central area of the triangles was 13.2% and 7.5% for the first and second datasets, respectively. As none of the datasets showed more than 30% of noise, all of them contained sufficient phylogenetic signal.

3.3. Phylogenetic Analysis

All new sequences were classified as subtype 1b by both Oxford and COMET subtyping tools, and by phylogenetic analysis. The ML phylogenetic tree of the first dataset showed that all the 53 sequences collected from the Calabria Region were in the same statistically supported clade, closely related to the references subtype 1b and were therefore classified as subtype 1b (Figure 1).

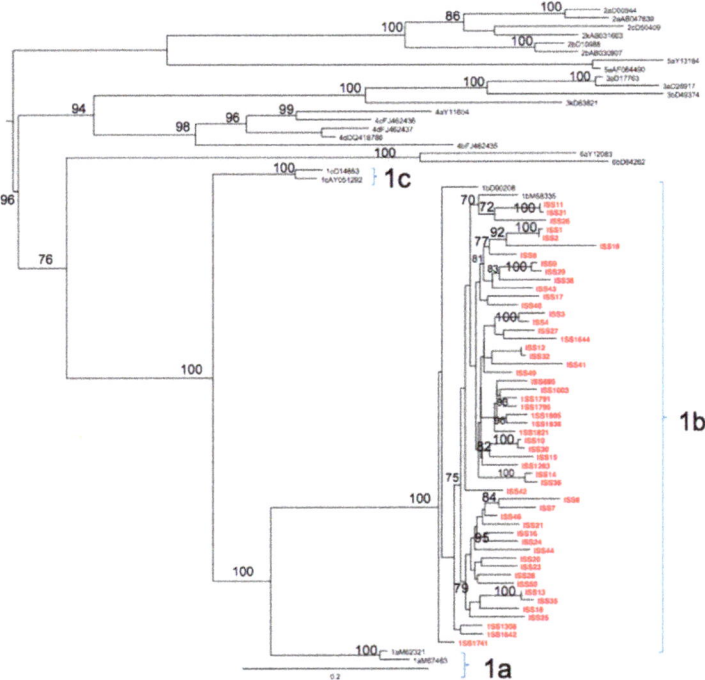

Figure 1. Maximum likelihood phylogenetic tree of the first HCV NS5B dataset. The tree was rooted by using the midpoint rooting method. Branch lengths were estimated with the best fitting nucleotide substitution model according to a hierarchical likelihood ratio test, and were drawn to scale with the bar at the bottom indicating 0.2 nucleotide substitutions per site. The values along a branch represent significant statistical support for the clade subtending that branch (bootstrap support >75%). The Italian (Calabria Region) sequences are highlighted in red. Clades 1b, 1c and 1a are also highlighted with brackets.

The maximum likelihood phylogenetic tree of the second dataset showed the presence of a supported cluster and a main statistically supported clade (Figure 2).

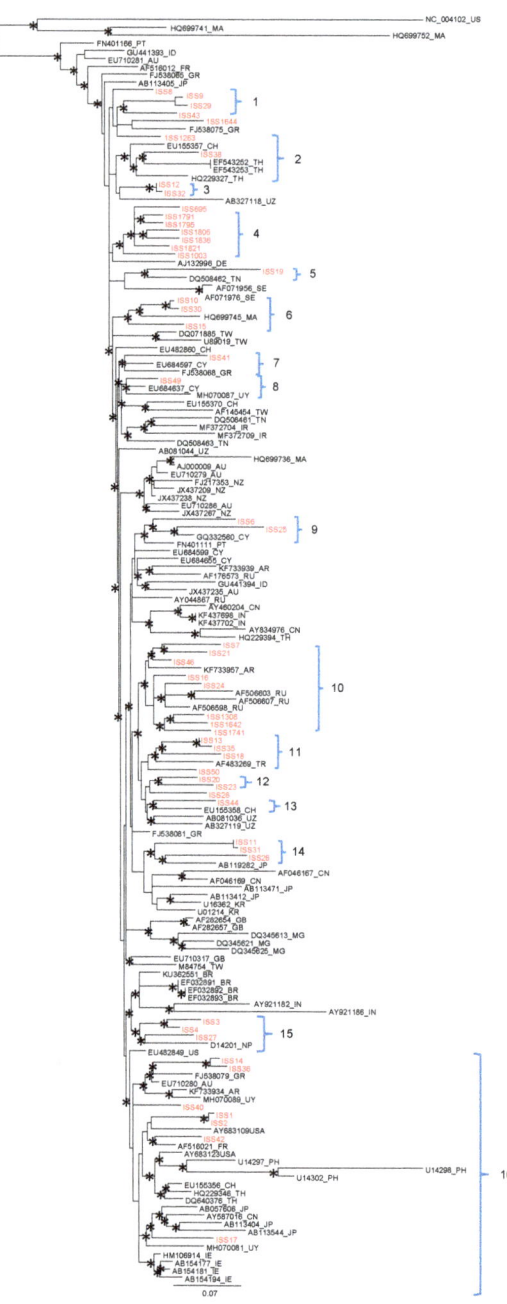

Figure 2. Maximum likelihood phylogenetic tree of the second dataset HCV1b dataset. The tree was rooted by using the midpoint rooting method. Branch lengths were estimated with the best fitting nucleotide substitution model according to a hierarchical likelihood ratio test, and were drawn to scale with the bar at the bottom indicating 0.07 nucleotide substitutions per site. The asterisk (*) along a branch represents significant statistical support for the clade subtending that branch (bootstrap support >75%). The main statistically significant sequences are highlighted with brackets.

The supported cluster included three foreign (Morocco and US) related sequences. Within the main clade, the HCV1b Italian (Calabria Region) sequences were distributed in 16 statistically supported clusters. Twelve clusters (12/16, 75%), presented foreign HCV 1b reference sequences intermixed with sequences from Italy (Clusters: 2, 5, 6, 7, 8, 9, 10, 11, 13, 14, 15, 16). Four statistically significant monophyletic clusters, including only sequences from Calabria were also observed (clusters: 1, 3, 4, 12).

Cluster 1 included three sequences from Catanzaro (ISS 9, 29, 43) reporting the following risk factors: blood transfusion/cohabitation, surgery/dental treatment and dental treatment, respectively.

The sequence ISS38 was located in cluster 2 with one reference from Switzerland and three from Thailand. Cluster 3 was composed of two Calabrian sequences (ISS 12 and 32) characterized respectively, by the following risk factors: dental treatment and blood transfusion/dental treatment. Interestingly, cluster 4 included seven sequences (ISS 695; 1791, 1795, 1805, 1836, 1821, 1003), closely related to each other, all from Sersale village. The following risk factors were reported: surgery, cohabitation with HCV positive, sharing glass syringes and blood transfusion (ISS 695), surgery and sharing glass syringes (ISS 1003, 1805, 1821, 1836), no risk factors (ISS 1791, 1795). Cluster 5 included one isolate from Calabria (Catanzaro) reporting blood transfusion as a risk factor and related to a sequence from Tunisia. Cluster 6 was composed of three isolates (ISS10, 30 and 15) from Catanzaro (risk factors: blood transfusion, surgery/dental treatment and surgery) related to a sequence from Morocco. Cluster 7 included one isolate (ISS 41) from Catanzaro characterized by the following risk factor: surgery, related to one reference from Cyprus and one from Greece. Cluster 8 included isolate ISS49 (risk factors: surgery and blood transfusion), one reference from Cyprus and one from Uruguay. Cluster 9 included two isolates from Catanzaro, ISS6 and ISS25 (risk factors: surgery/multiple blood transfusion and surgery/dental treatment, respectively) related to a sequence from Cyprus and another from Portugal. Cluster 10 included eight isolates from Calabria (ISS 7, 21, 46, 16, 24, 1308, 164, 1741), three of which from Sersale, related to one reference from Argentina and three from Russia. Cluster 11 was characterized by three sequences from Catanzaro (ISS 13, 35 and 18) reporting the following risk factors (surgery, surgery/dental treatment, dental treatment, respectively) and related to a reference from Turkey. Cluster 12 included two isolates collected from Catanzaro (ISS 20 and 23) with risk factors: surgery/blood transfusion and surgery/dental treatment, respectively. Cluster 13 was composed of two sequences, the isolate ISS 44 from Catanzaro (reporting surgery/cohabitation as risk factors) related to a reference from Switzerland. Cluster 14 included three isolates from Catanzaro (ISS 11, 31 and 26) reporting the following risk factors (dental treatment, surgery, blood transfusion, and cohabitation) related to a reference from Japan. Cluster 15 included three sequences (ISS 3, 4 and 27) characterized by the following risk factors: surgery/dental treatment; surgery/blood transfusion; surgery/dental treatment/cohabitation and related to a reference from Nepal. Cluster 16 included seven isolates from Catanzaro (ISS 14, 36, 40, 1, 2, 42, 17) intermixed with many sequences sampled from different countries: USA, Greece, Austria, Argentina, Uruguay, France, Philippines, Switzerland, Thailand, Japan, China and Ireland.

3.4. Substitutions on Target Regions in Patients Naïve to DAA

The total (100%) of NS5B amplicons were sequenced. Nine (40%) NS5A amplicons were not successfully sequenced, while 10 sequences were not of suitable length for RAS screening. Available NS5A and NS5B sequences at the time of genotyping were screened for RASs and nonsynonymous substitutions. We identified the L159F NS5B substitution, conferring resistance to sofosbuvir (SOF), in 15/41 (ISS 6, 7, 13, 16, 18, 20, 21, 23, 24, 25, 28, 35, 44, 46, 50) isolates, among them 8/15 (ISS 6, 13, 21, 24, 25, 28, 35, 46) also carried the C316N NS5B related to dasabuvir resistance. In particular, frequency of detected NS5B RASs was 36.6%, while frequency of RASs carried on NS5A region was 22.7%.

The Y93H, associated with resistance to daclatasvir, elbasvir, ledipasvir (LPV), ombitasvir (OMV) and pibrentasvir was detected on NS5A in 3/22 (ISS 16, 24, 30) isolates. The

L31M substitution associated with resistance to all drugs mentioned above plus velpatasvir was found in 1/22 (ISS 21) isolate. Interestingly, all three isolates carried Y93H plus K108R substitution. The A92T NS5A OMV and LPV associated resistance was detected in 1/22 (ISS 2) isolate. Among patients who reported RASs in the viral population, seven have been previously treated with an IFN regimen with or without RBV and were classified as non-responders (4/7) or relapsers (3/7) with liver stiffness F3 or F4. On the other hand, the 33.3% of patients without RASs were IFN experienced with or without RBV. The median baseline RNA viral load was 2,280,000 IU/mL.

4. Discussion

In order to explore the spread of HCV1b in the Calabria Region, we analyzed NS5B population sequences, obtained from two cohorts of positive individuals, enrolled in different time spans, using phylogenetic analysis. In addition, viral isolates collected between 2015 and 2016 from naïve and IFN/pegIFN-α/RBV treated patients were analyzed in the NS5B and NS5A regions to assess the presence of RASs with the potential to impact on DAA therapy.

Molecular analysis was carried out on 53 sequences of HCV subtype 1b, previously characterized by Inno-Lipa and confirmed by sequencing analysis. As reported in previous studies, subtype 1b, together with subtype 2c, are the most prevalent genotypes in Italy followed by genotypes 3 and 4 [3,6]. HCV1b diffusion worldwide is related to several risk factors, such as blood transfusions, dental treatment, unsafe reuse of nondisposable syringes [27,28]. In previous studies, transmission of two subtypes was already correlated to specific risk factors in the Calabria Region. HCV4d was found related to intravenous drug use and blood transfusion, while HCV2c infection was maintained by unsafe use of glass syringes followed by surgery and unsafe blood transfusion [29,30].

In this work, we investigated possible transmission patterns in a regionally representative sample from a small village (Sersale), where a seminal HCV prevalence study was conducted, and a metropolitan area of the Calabria region [13]. The ML phylogenetic tree shows that the HCV1b Calabria sequences were distributed in 16 statistically supported clusters. Twelve clusters (75%), contained Italian sequences mixed with foreign HCV1b references while four statistically significant monophyletic clusters included only sequences from Calabria (clusters: 1, 3, 4, 12). In particular, cluster 4 contained only seven closely related Italian sequences collected from Sersale village.

In this study, the majority (58.5%) of the enrolled individuals reported multiple risk factors, most of which were surgical intervention and dental treatment (n = 8) or surgical intervention and glass syringes (n = 7). Individually, we observed that the most frequent risk factors were dental treatment (16.9%) and surgical intervention (13.2%). Interestingly, the risk factors for HCV acquisition in cluster 4 were medical interventions and multiple use of glass syringes in a family setting as reported in 71% (no. 5/7) of patients (ISS 695, 1003, 1805, 1821, 1836).

Our analysis indicates that in the past, subtype 1b was maintained, by sporadic infections, mainly acquired through unsafe use of glass syringes especially in some limited areas of southern Italy, such as Sersale, a small town located 30 miles from Catanzaro. Conversely, in the metropolitan area, other transmission routes, such as dental treatment and surgical intervention had a significant influence on the dissemination of HCV subtype 1b throughout the Calabria Region. Interestingly, a community-based survey in the Calabria Region, revealed a high percentage of possible risk factors for HCV acquisition, such as dental treatment (69.5%) and glass syringes injections (25.8%) [31].

On the other hand, DAA treatment of hepatitis C could be influenced by baseline RASs naturally occurring in the viral genome [25,32]. It has been reported that 3% of HCV positive patients have no virological response, due to the presence of comorbidities and/or RASs in viral isolates, especially in the NS5A viral region [33]. We detected NS5B L159F alone in 15/41 (36.5%) and in association with C316N in 8/41 (19.5%) patients, respectively. This last substitution, showing a global frequency of 31.4% in HCV1b, is now defined as a fitness-associated substitution when combined with the L159F [34]. Therefore, both amino acid variants were associated with a lower response to SOF [35]. Interestingly, NS5B S282T conferring high-level resistance to SOF-containing regimens, was not detected among our isolates, despite being present in 99.1% of worldwide strains [25]. In three patients, NS5A sequences carried the Y93H substitution, currently the major clinically relevant RAS contributing to failure of many approved IFN-free regimens [36]. Additionally, all three isolates showed the Y93H + K108R profile, which is associated with a minor affinity to OMV drug with respect to the Y93H + R108K combination as previously reported [37]. However, the 97% of treated patients with DAAs achieved sustained virological response (SVR). According to our experience about a single-center cohort in Southern Italy, the SVR rate was 97% for the older age group, 96% for people under 65 years old, finally 94% and 100% for cirrhotic and non-cirrhotic patients, respectively [38].

5. Conclusions

Despite the sample size being a limitation of the study, this suggests that the spread of HCV1b was maintained in the Calabria Region by sporadic infections, mainly acquired through the unsafe use of glass syringes, dental treatment and surgical intervention. Even if our analysis was performed on samples collected in 2015–2016, the frequency of natural RASs carried on subtype-specific viral strains, as well as comorbidities of treated patients, should be taken into account for the effectiveness of IFN-free regimens to eradicate HCV infection.

Supplementary Materials: The following are available online at https://www.mdpi.com/article/10.3390/jcm10081655/s1, Figure S1: Likelihood mapping of HCV NS5B first (a) and second (b) dataset.

Author Contributions: A.R.C. and R.B.: conceptualization. A.C., S.T., M.E., A.L.P., G.P., G.S.B., A.Q., G.M.: methodology. A.C., S.T., M.E., A.L.P., G.P., N.M.: A.C., S.T., M.E., G.P.: formal analysis. investigation. E.M.T., C.C., M.M., F.S., C.T.: data curation. A.C., S.T., A.L.P., N.M.: writing—original draft preparation. A.R.C., M.C.L., C.T., N.M.: writing—review and editing. A.R.C.: supervision. All authors have read and agreed to the published version of the manuscript.

Funding: This research received no external funding.

Institutional Review Board Statement: The study was conducted according to the guidelines of the Declaration of Helsinki, and approved by the Ethical Committee (#100; 27 April 2017) of the "Mater Domini" University Teaching Hospital of Catanzaro, Italy.

Informed Consent Statement: Patient consent was waived due to non-interventional study. The Ethical Committee approved the criteria that there is no need for informed consent for a non-interventional study.

Data Availability Statement: The 41 NS5B and 22 NS5A newly generated sequences used for molecular analysis have been uploaded to GenBank under the following accession numbers: MW357752-MW357814. Materials supporting the findings of this study are available within the article.

Acknowledgments: The authors would like to thank Neill J. Adams (Department of Health Sciences, Institute of Microbiology, "Magna Grecia" University of Catanzaro, Italy) who checked the English throughout the manuscript. Maria Mazzitelli was supported as PhD student by European Commission (FESR FSE 2014-2020) and by Calabria Region (Italy). European Commission and Calabria Region cannot be held responsible for any use, which may be made of information contained therein.

Conflicts of Interest: The authors declare no conflict of interest.

References

1. European Association for the Study of the Liver. EASL Recommendations on Treatment of Hepatitis C 2020. *J. Hepatol.* **2020**, *73*, 1170–1218.
2. Borgia, S.M.; Hedskog, C.; Parhy, B.; Hyland, R.H.; Stamm, L.M.; Brainard, D.M.; Subramanian, M.G.; McHutchison, J.G.; Mo, H.; Svarovskaia, E.; et al. Identification of a Novel Hepatitis C Virus Genotype From Punjab, India: Expanding Classification of Hepatitis C Virus Into 8 Genotypes. *J. Infect. Dis.* **2018**, *218*, 1722–1729. [CrossRef]

3. Marascio, N.; Liberto, M.C.; Barreca, G.S.; Zicca, E.; Quirino, A.; Lamberti, A.G.; Bianco, G.; Matera, G.; Surace, L.; Berardelli, G.; et al. Update on epidemiology of HCV in Italy: Focus on the Calabria Region. *BMC Infect. Dis.* **2014**, *14*, S2. [CrossRef] [PubMed]
4. Kartashev, V.; Döring, M.; Nieto, L.; Coletta, E.; Kaiser, R.; Sierra, S.; Guerrero, A.; Stoiber, H.; Paar, C.; Vandamme, A.; et al. New findings in HCV genotype distribution in selected West European, Russian and Israeli regions. *J. Clin. Virol.* **2016**, *81*, 82–89. [CrossRef] [PubMed]
5. Magiorkinis, G.; Magiorkinis, E.; Paraskevis, D.; Ho, S.Y.W.; Shapiro, B.; Pybus, O.G.; Allain, J.-P.; Hatzakis, A. The Global Spread of Hepatitis C Virus 1a and 1b: A Phylodynamic and Phylogeographic Analysis. *PLoS Med.* **2009**, *6*, e1000198. [CrossRef]
6. Ansaldi, F.; Bruzzone, B.; Salmaso, S.; Rota, M.C.; Durando, P.; Gasparini, R.; Icardi, G. Different seroprevalence and molecular epidemiology patterns of hepatitis C virus infection in Italy. *J. Med. Virol.* **2005**, *76*, 327–332. [CrossRef] [PubMed]
7. Mitra, A.K. Hepatitis C-related hepatocellular carcinoma: Prevalence around the world, factors interacting, and role of genotypes. *Epidemiol. Rev.* **1999**, *21*, 180–187. [CrossRef] [PubMed]
8. Liberto, M.C.; Marascio, N.; Zicca, E.; Matera, G. Epidemiological features and specificities of HCV infection: A hospital-based cohort study in a university medical center of Calabria region. *BMC Infect. Dis.* **2012**, *12*, S4. [CrossRef]
9. Cuypers, L.; Snoeck, J.; Vrancken, B.; Kerremans, L.; Vuagniaux, G.; Verbeeck, J.; Nevens, F.; Camacho, R.J.; Vandamme, A.M.; Van Dooren, S. A near-full length genotypic assay for HCV1b. *J. Virol. Methods* **2014**, *209*, 126–135. [CrossRef]
10. Marascio, N.; Quirino, A.; Barreca, G.S.; Galati, L.; Costa, C.; Pisani, V.; Mazzitelli, M.; Matera, G.; Liberto, M.C.; Focà, A.; et al. Discussion on critical points for a tailored therapy to cure hepatitis C virus infection. *Clin. Mol. Hepatol.* **2019**, *25*, 30–36. [CrossRef]
11. Torti, C.; Zazzi, M.; Abenavoli, L.; Trapasso, F.; Cesario, F.; Corigliano, D.; Cosco, L.; Costa, C.; Curia, R.L.; De Rosa, M.; et al. SINERGIE Study Group. Future research and collaboration: The "SINERGIE" project on HCV (South Italian Network for Rational Guidelines and International Epidemiology). *BMC Infect. Dis.* **2012**, *12*, S9. [CrossRef] [PubMed]
12. Marascio, N.; Mazzitelli, M.; Scarlata, G.G.M.; Giancotti, A.; Barreca, G.S.; Lamberti, A.G.; Divenuto, F.; Costa, C.; Trecarichi, E.M.; Matera, G.; et al. HCV Antibody Prevalence and Genotype Evolution in a Teaching Hospital, Calabria Region, Southern Italy Over A Decade (2008–2018). *Open Microbiol.* **2020**, *14*, 84–90. [CrossRef]
13. Guadagnino, V.; Stroffolini, T.; Caroleo, B.; Menniti Ippolito, F.; Rapicetta, M.; Ciccaglione, A.R.; Chionne, P.; Madonna, E.; Costantino, A.; De Sarro, G.; et al. Hepatitis C virus infection in an endemic area of Southern Italy 14 years later: Evidence for a vanishing infection. *Dig. Liver Dis.* **2013**, *45*, 403–407. [CrossRef] [PubMed]
14. Castera, L.; Vergniol, J.; Foucher, J.; Le Bail, B.; Chanteloup, E.; Haaser, M.; Darriet, M.; Couzigou, P.; de Ledinghen, V. Prospective comparison of transient elastography, Fibrotest, APRI, and liver biopsy for the assessment of fibrosis in chronic hepatitis C. *Gastroenterology* **2005**, *128*, 343–350. [CrossRef]
15. Pybus, O.G.; Barnes, E.; Taggart, R.; Lemey, P.; Markov, P.V.; Rasachak, B.; Syhavong, B.; Phetsouvanah, R.; Sheridan, I.; Humphreys, I.S.; et al. Genetic history of hepatitis C virus in East Asia. *J. Virol.* **2009**, *83*, 1071–1082. [CrossRef]
16. Lindström, I.; Kjellin, M.; Palanisamy, N.; Bondeson, K.; Wesslén, L.; Lannergard, A.; Lennerstrand, J. Prevalence of polymorphisms with significant resistance to NS5A inhibitors in treatment-naive patients with hepatitis C virus genotypes 1a and 3a in Sweden. *Infect. Dis.* **2015**, *47*, 555–562. [CrossRef]
17. Katoh, K.; Standley, D.M. MAFFT multiple sequence alignment software version 7: Improvements in performance and usability. *Mol. Biol. Evol.* **2013**, *30*, 772–780. [CrossRef]
18. Afgan, E.; Baker, D.; Batut, B.; van den Beek, M.; Bouvier, D.; Cech, M.; Chilton, J.; Clements, D.; Coraor, N.; Grüning, B.A.; et al. The Galaxy platform for accessible, reproducible and collaborative biomedical analyses: 2018 update. *Nucleic Acids Res.* **2018**, *46*, W537–W544. Available online: https://usegalaxy.org/ (accessed on 27 March 2020). [CrossRef]
19. Hall, T.A. BioEdit: A User-Friendly Biological Sequence Alignment Editor and Analysis Program for Windows 95/98/NT. *Nucleic Acids Symp. Ser.* **1999**, *41*, 95–98.
20. de Oliveira, T.; Deforche, K.; Cassol, S.; Salminen, M.; Paraskevis, D.; Seebregts, C.; Snoeck, J.; van Rensburg, E.J.; Wensing, A.M.; van de Vijver, D.A.; et al. An automated genotyping system for analysis of HIV-1 and other microbial sequences. *Bioinformatics* **2005**, *21*, 3797–3800. Available online: http://dbpartners.stanford.edu/RegaSubtyping/html/subtypinghcvSUB.html (accessed on 20 April 2020). [CrossRef]
21. Struck, D.; Lawyer, G.; Ternes, A.M.; Schmit, J.C.; Perez Bercoff, D. COMET: Adaptive context-based modeling for ultrafast HIV-1 subtype identification. *Nucleic Acids Res.* **2014**, *42*, e144. Available online: https://comet.lih.lu/index.php?cat=hcv (accessed on 20 April 2020). [CrossRef]
22. Schmidt, H.A.; Strimmer, K.; Vingron, M.; von Haeseler, A. TREE-PUZZLE: Maximum likelihood phylogenetic analysis using quartets and parallel computing. *Bioinformatics* **2002**, *18*, 502–504. [CrossRef]
23. Nguyen, L.T.; Schmidt, H.A.; von Haeseler, A.; Minh, B.Q. IQ-TREE: A fast and effective stochastic algorithm for estimating maximum likelihood phylogenies. *Mol. Biol. Evol.* **2015**, *32*, 268–274. [CrossRef]
24. Kalaghatgi, P.; Sikorski, A.M.; Knops, E.; Rupp, D.; Sierra, S.; Heger, E.; Neumann-Fraune, M.; Beggel, B.; Walker, A.; Timm, J.; et al. Geno2pheno[HCV]—A web-based interpretation system to support hepatitis C treatment decisions in the era of direct-acting antiviral agents. *PLoS ONE* **2016**, *11*, 1416. [CrossRef] [PubMed]
25. Di Maio, V.C.; Cento, V.; Lenci, I.; Aragri, M.; Rossi, P.; Barbaliscia, S.; Melis, M.; Verucchi, G.; Magni, C.F.; Teti, E.; et al. HCV Italian Resistance Network Study Group. Multiclass HCV resistance to direct-acting antiviral failure in real-life patients advocates for tailored second-line therapies. *Liver Int.* **2017**, *37*, 514–528. [CrossRef]

26. Benson, D.A.; Clark, K.; Karsch-Mizrachi, I.; Lipman, D.J.; Ostell, J.; Sayers, E.W. GenBank. *Nucleic Acids Res.* **2014**, *42*, 32–37. [CrossRef] [PubMed]
27. Alter, M.J. HCV routes of transmission: What goes around comes around. *Semin. Liver Dis.* **2011**, *31*, 340–346. [CrossRef] [PubMed]
28. Olmstead, A.D.; Joy, J.B.; Montoya, V.; Luo, I.; Poon, A.F.; Jacka, B.; Lamoury, F.; Applegate, T.; Montaner, J.; Khudyakov, Y.; et al. A molecular phylogenetics-based approach for identifying recent hepatitis C virus transmission events. *Infect. Genet. Evol.* **2015**, *33*, 101–109. [CrossRef]
29. Ciccozzi, M.; Equestre, M.; Costantino, A.; Marascio, N.; Quirino, A.; Lo Presti, A.; Cella, E.; Bruni, R.; Liberto, M.C.; Focà, A.; et al. Hepatitis C virus genotype 4d in Southern Italy: Reconstruction of its origin and spread by a phylodynamic analysis. *J. Med. Virol.* **2012**, *84*, 1613–1619. [CrossRef]
30. Marascio, N.; Ciccozzi, M.; Equestre, M.; Lo Presti, A.; Costantino, A.; Cella, E.; Bruni, R.; Liberto, M.C.; Pisani, G.; Zicca, E.; et al. Back to the origin of HCV 2c subtype and spreading to the Calabria region (Southern Italy) over the last two centuries: A phylogenetic study. *Infect. Genet. Evol.* **2014**, *26*, 352–358. [CrossRef]
31. Serraino, R.; Mazzitelli, M.; Greco, G.; Serapide, F.; Scaglione, V.; Marascio, N.; Trecarichi, E.M.; Torti, C. Risk factors for hepatitis B and C among healthy population: A community-based survey from four districts of Southern Italy. *Infez. Med.* **2020**, *28*, 223–226.
32. Marascio, N.; Pavia, G.; Strazzulla, A.; Dierckx, T.; Cuypers, L.; Vrancken, B.; Barreca, G.S.; Mirante, T.; Malanga, D.; Oliveira, D.M.; et al. The SINERGIE-UMG Study Group. Detection of Natural Resistance-Associated Substitutions by Ion Semiconductor Technology in HCV1b Positive, Direct-Acting Antiviral Agents-Naïve Patients. *Int. J. Mol. Sci.* **2016**, *17*, 1416. [CrossRef]
33. Calvaruso, V.; Petta, S.; Craxì, A. Is global elimination of HCV realistic? *Liver Int.* **2018**, *38*, 40–46. [CrossRef] [PubMed]
34. Cuypers, L.; Li, G.; Libin, P.; Piampongsant, S.; Vandamme, A.M.; Theys, K. Genetic Diversity and Selective Pressure in Hepatitis C Virus Genotypes 1–6: Significance for Direct-Acting Antiviral Treatment and Drug Resistance. *Viruses* **2015**, *7*, 5018–5039. [CrossRef] [PubMed]
35. Gaspareto, K.V.; Ribeiro, R.M.; de Mello Malta, F.; Gomes-Gouvêa, M.S.; Muto, N.H.; Romano, C.M.; Mendes-Correa, M.C.; Carrilho, F.J.; Sabino, E.C.; Rebello Pinho, J.R. Resistance-associated variants in HCV subtypes 1a and 1b detected by Ion Torrent sequencing platform. *Antivir. Ther.* **2016**, *21*, 653–660. [CrossRef] [PubMed]
36. Zeuzem, S.; Mizokami, M.; Pianko, S.; Mangia, A.; Han, K.H.; Martin, R.; Svarovskaia, E.; Dvory-Sobol, H.; Doehle, B.; Hedskog, C.; et al. NS5A resistance-associated substitutions in patients with genotype 1 hepatitis C virus: Prevalence and effect on treatment outcome. *J. Hepatol.* **2017**, *66*, 910–918. [CrossRef] [PubMed]
37. Marascio, N.; Pavia, G.; Romeo, I.; Talarico, C.; Di Salvo, S.; Reale, M.; Marano, V.; Barreca, G.S.; Fabiani, F.; Perrotti, N.; et al. Real-life 3D therapy failure: Analysis of NS5A 93H RAS plus 108 K polymorphism in complex with ombitasvir by molecular modeling. *J. Med. Virol.* **2018**, *90*, 1257–1263. [CrossRef]
38. Scaglione, V.; Mazzitelli, M.; Costa, C.; Pisani, V.; Greco, G.; Serapide, F.; Lionello, R.; La Gamba, V.; Marascio, N.; Trecarichi, E.M.; et al. Virological and Clinical Outcome of DAA Containing Regimens in a Cohort of Patients in Calabria Region (Southern Italy). *Medicina* **2020**, *56*, 101. [CrossRef]

Review

Noninvasive Assessment of Hepatitis C Virus Infected Patients Using Vibration-Controlled Transient Elastography

Mira Florea [1,†], Teodora Serban [2,†], George Razvan Tirpe [3,‡], Alexandru Tirpe [4,‡] and Monica Lupsor-Platon [2,5,*]

1. Community Medicine Department, Iuliu Hatieganu University of Medicine and Pharmacy, 400012 Cluj-Napoca, Romania; miraflorea@umfcluj.ro
2. Medical Imaging Department, Iuliu Hatieganu University of Medicine and Pharmacy, 400012 Cluj-Napoca, Romania; serban.teodora8@gmail.com
3. Department of Radiology and Medical Imaging, County Emergency Hospital Cluj-Napoca, 3-5 Clinicilor Street, 400000 Cluj-Napoca, Romania; razvantirpe@gmail.com
4. Research Center for Functional Genomics, Biomedicine and Translational Medicine, Iuliu Hatieganu University of Medicine and Pharmacy, 23 Marinescu Street, 400337 Cluj-Napoca, Romania; altirpe@gmail.com
5. Medical Imaging Department, Regional Institute of Gastroenterology and Hepatology, 400162 Cluj-Napoca, Romania
* Correspondence: monica.lupsor@umfcluj.ro
† M.F. and T.S. share the first co-authorship.
‡ These authors have equal contribution to the work.

Abstract: Chronic infection with hepatitis C virus (HCV) is one of the leading causes of cirrhosis and hepatocellular carcinoma (HCC). Surveillance of these patients is an essential strategy in the prevention chain, including in the pre/post-antiviral treatment states. Ultrasound elastography techniques are emerging as key methods in the assessment of liver diseases, with a number of advantages such as their rapid, noninvasive, and cost-effective characters. The present paper critically reviews the performance of vibration-controlled transient elastography (VCTE) in the assessment of HCV patients. VCTE measures liver stiffness (LS) and the ultrasonic attenuation through the embedded controlled attenuation parameter (CAP), providing the clinician with a tool for assessing fibrosis, cirrhosis, and steatosis in a noninvasive manner. Moreover, standardized LS values enable proper staging of the underlying fibrosis, leading to an accurate identification of a subset of HCV patients that present a high risk for complications. In addition, VCTE is a valuable technique in evaluating liver fibrosis prior to HCV therapy. However, its applicability in monitoring fibrosis regression after HCV eradication is currently limited and further studies should focus on extending the boundaries of VCTE in this context. From a different perspective, VCTE may be effective in identifying clinically significant portal hypertension (CSPH). An emerging prospect of clinical significance that warrants further study is the identification of esophageal varices. Our opinion is that the advantages of VCTE currently outweigh those of other surveillance methods.

Keywords: chronic hepatitis C; vibration controlled transient elastography; fibrosis; steatosis; hepatocellular carcinoma

1. Introduction

The global estimates of hepatitis C virus (HCV) infection appraised chronic hepatitis C (CHC) as one of the leading causes of cirrhosis and hepatocellular carcinoma (HCC), with an approximate global prevalence of HCV infection at 1.6% [1,2]. Specifically, CHC patients may silently develop cirrhosis in up to 20% of cases. In addition, patients with CHC and cirrhosis may develop HCC in up to 5% of cases per year [3]. HCV transmission routes are dependent on blood and blood products [4]. The diagnosis of HCV infection can be achieved through serologic assays and molecular RNA-based assays. In general terms, third generation serologic assays have a sensitivity of over 99% when CHC is suspected [4]. However, the silent progression of CHC towards cirrhosis prompts for new diagnostic means that can identify this pathological tendency early on the evolution axis. Liver fibrosis (LF) staging is paramount as it carries multiple roles—it is essential for the antiviral therapy, in the management of individuals after successful HCV treatment, and for prognosis purposes [5]. In addition, steatosis can accelerate liver fibrosis progression in HCV patients, and is associated with lower virologic response to antiviral therapy [6]. Although there is evidence of the contribution of ultrasound and even of artificial intelligence-enhanced US image analysis in steatosis quantification [7], new imaging techniques such as elastography are considered an essential add-on. The highly efficient direct-acting antiviral (DAA) therapies and noninvasive measures of liver fibrosis are two scientific advances that changed the management of patients with chronic HCV infection in the last decade [8].

Liver biopsy (LB) is an invasive method for staging fibrosis and grading steatosis and necroinflammatory activity [1]. It presents a number of drawbacks, including the risk of serious complications that may influence the patient acceptance rate and the lack of dynamic evaluation of liver fibrosis in time [9,10]. Although LB remains the reference standard for assessing necroinflammation and fibrosis, its limitations as an invasive procedure and requires repeated sampling, which has led to the use and development of several other noninvasive test as alternatives [11].

Conventional ultrasonography (US) (with or without contrast enhancement) is a noninvasive, cost-effective, widely available, and rapid technique that enables the examination of patients with chronic liver diseases (CLD) [12]. By evaluating structural changes, US proved to be particularly useful for the detection of cirrhosis and focal liver lesions (FLL) [12,13]. However, US fails to discern between lower stages of fibrosis, in which has led to the introduction of US elastography in order to overcome this drawback [14].

Vibration-controlled transient elastography (VCTE) is a novel, noninvasive, cost-efficient method for fibrosis staging using liver stiffness measurement (LSM) [10]. Furthermore, through the embedded Controlled Attenuation Parameter (CAP) tool, VCTE is able to simultaneously assess liver steatosis by estimating the total ultrasonic attenuation [15]. The current tendency of liver fibrosis assessment leans in favor of VCTE, as ultrasound elastography methods are becoming the standard of care in comparison to liver biopsy [1].

The present review aims to explore the current status of VCTE as noninvasive imaging assessment tool of HCV-infected patients through the lens of evidence-based medicine, underlining the differences between VCTE and conventional US.

2. The Principle of Vibration-Controlled Transient Elastography (VCTE, TE)

As previously mentioned, VCTE is a quantitative method for the noninvasive assessment of liver stiffness. It is composed of a device with readout—FibroScan® (Echosens, Paris, France)—and different types of probes (S, M and XL). Choosing the correct transducer, according to the circumference of the patients' thorax, is an important step in order to have a successful examination. While a circumference lower than 75 cm indicates the use of the S probe, the M probe is indicated for a circumference of over 75 cm. Furthermore, if the distance between the skin and liver capsule is greater than 25 mm, the XL transducer is the preferred option. It is worth mentioning that the median liver stiffness is significantly lower with XL probe compared to the M probe [16].

The ideal VCTE examination takes place with a patient who has fasted for 3 h prior to the measurement [17,18]. Depending on the thickness of the abdominal wall, one of the handheld probes is chosen and, together with the applied conduction gel, the probe is placed intercostally overlying the right hepatic lobe [19–21]. The probe generates a vibration wave, which travels through the liver and simultaneously receives ultrasound waves, calculating liver stiffness, rendered in kilopascal (kPa). In order to provide a median value of LS, ten successful measurements are required. LS can range widely between 2.5–75 kPa, with normal values being around 5 kPa. LS does not absolutely stage fibrosis like a biopsy would, but high values are significantly correlated with histology and are able to provide a risk estimate for advanced liver disease [22].

Simultaneously, the CAP (measured in dB/m) is calculated based on the attenuation of the ultrasound signal, with the purpose of evaluating the underlying liver steatosis in a noninvasive manner [23]. Chon et al. [24] suggested that the range of normal CAP values within the 5th–95th percentiles was 156.0–287.8 dB/m, with gender, body mass index, diabetes, and etiology independently affecting CAP values [25].

3. Pathological Changes Influencing Liver Stiffness

A comprehensive evaluation of the factors that increase liver stiffness is considered paramount. In a study by Lupsor et al. [26] that included 324 HCV patients, the authors found a strong correlation between LS and different histopathological parameters such as fibrosis ($r = 0.759$, $p < 0.0005$), necroinflammatory activity ($r = 0.378$, $p < 0.0005$), and steatosis ($r = 0.255$, $p < 0.0005$). Among these three, however, the stage of fibrosis is the single most important predictor.

Nevertheless, ingestion of food prior to LS measurement is another reason for increased kPa values. In a study by Arena et al. [17], LS was evaluated following a standardized meal in 125 confirmed HCV patients at different stages of fibrotic evolution. An elevation in kPa values was observed 15 to 45 minutes after ingestion of the meal and was higher among patients with increased stages of fibrosis ($p < 0.001$) and maximal among those with cirrhosis. Other factors that influence liver stiffness irrespective of fibrosis are mechanic cholestasis, central venous pressure and congestion, portal or arterial pressure, alcohol consumption, water retention, Valsalva and orthostatic maneuvers, as well as amyloidosis [27,28].

A rise in LS values along with a rise in ALT levels can be detected in patients with hepatitis due to cellular swelling and cholestasis. Furthermore, the increased stiffness values identified in patients with relapsed chronic hepatitis are not only found due to fibrosis, but also due to the superimposed cellular intumescence [29]. In a study by Bota et al. [30], the LS cutoffs were significantly higher in patients with increased ALT levels between 1.1 and 5-fold the standard value compared to those with normal ALT levels, 12.3 kPa versus 9.1 kPa, respectively. Consequently, caution must be taken when assessing liver stiffness in patients with increased ALT values because there is a risk of overestimating the stage of fibrosis [16].

4. Fibrosis Assessment by VCTE in HCV-Infected Patients

Among patients with CHC, determining liver fibrosis stage is essential for prognosis, follow-up, and antiviral therapy [5]. The European Federation of Societies for Ultrasound in Medicine and Biology (EFSUMB) guidelines outline that the two clinically relevant endpoints in HCV patients are the detection of significant fibrosis and, above anything else, the detection of cirrhosis [27]

As previously implied, the widely available US method fails to discern fibrosis in its early stages, which led to the introduction of novel elastography technologies. In fact, a recent study by Zhang et al. [13] found VCTE to be superior to US for the detection of significant fibrosis (AUROC, 0.84 versus 0.73; $p = 0.02$), advanced fibrosis (AUROC, 0.95 versus 0.76; $p < 0.001$), and cirrhosis (AUROC, 0.96 versus 0.71; $p < 0.001$) in a cohort of 94 patients with chronic hepatitis B and nonalcoholic fatty liver disease. In addition, the combination of VCTE and US did not increase the diagnostic accuracy for neither of these stages, compared to VCTE alone. However, their association significantly improved the specificity (95.7% versus 76.6%, $p < 0.001$) and positive predictive value (94.3% versus 77.1%, $p = 0.002$) in contrast to VCTE alone. Similar results were observed by Wang et al. [31] in 320 patients with chronic viral hepatitis. Regarding other noninvasive methods, an evidence-based analysis concluded that neither FibroTest, nor acoustic radiation force impulse were superior to VCTE [32].

HCV infected patients are the first to have benefited from VCTE. Several studies reported excellent diagnostic accuracy of VCTE for the detection of fibrosis in HCV patients. As exemplified in Table 1, LS significantly correlates with the degree of liver fibrosis assessed by LB, even if some adjacent stages tend to overlap [10,26,33–43]. The AUROC values range from 0.838 to 0.936 for incipient fibrosis ($\geq$F1), 0.690 to 0.91 for significant fibrosis ($\geq$F2), 0.737 to 0.99 for advanced fibrosis ($\geq$F3), and 0.852 to 0.99 for cirrhosis (F4) prediction, at cutoff values of 5.3–5.5 kPa ($\geq$F1), 4.5–8.8 kPa ($\geq$F2), 9.1–11 kPa ($\geq$F3) and 11.3–16.9 kPa (F4), respectively. These values range significantly, mainly because of the varying prevalence of fibrosis stage in each study group along with the particular diagnostic aims of the investigation [44]. Thereby, the already defined cutoff values may not be applicable in all groups of patients, with different prevalence of fibrosis or diagnostic purposes [16].

Table 1. Performance of LS cutoff values by VCTE for predicting moderate fibrosis (≥F1), significant fibrosis (≥F2), advanced fibrosis (≥F3), and cirrhosis (F4) in chronic HCV infected patients.

Fibrosis Stage	≥F1			≥F2			≥F3			F4		
Study	Cutoff (kPa)	AUROC	Se/Sp (%)	Cutoff (kPa)	AUROC	Se/Sp (%)	Cutoff (kPa)	AUROC	Se/Sp (%)	Cutoff (kPa)	AUROC	Se/Sp (%)
Castera et al. [35] (n = 183)	N/S	N/S	N/S	7.1	0.83	67/89	9.5	0.90	73/91	12.5	0.95	87/91
Carrion et al. [45] (n = 169)	N/S	N/S	N/S	8.50	0.90	90/81	N/S	0.93	N/S	12.50	0.98	100/87
Ziol et al. [34] (n = 327) [1]	N/S	N/S	N/S	8.80	0.79/0.81	56/91	9.60	0.91/0.95	86/85	14.60	0.97/0.99	86/96
De Ledinghen et al. [36] (n = 77) [2]	N/S	N/S	N/S	4.5	0.72	93.2/17.9	N/S	N/S	N/S	11.8	0.97	100/92.7
Arena et al. [37] (n = 161)	N/S	N/S	N/S	7.8	0.91	83/82	10.8	0.99	91/94	14.8	0.98	94/92
Sporea et al. [46] (n = 191)	N/S	N/S	N/S	6.8	0.733	59.6/93.3	N/S	N/S	N/S	N/S	N/S	N/S
Nitta et al. [43] (n = 165)	N/S	N/S	N/S	7.1	0.87	80.8/80.3	9.6	0.91	87.7/82.4	11.6-16.9	0.93	62.5-91.7/78.9-91.5
Sanchez-Conde et al. [42] (n = 100)	N/S	N/S	N/S	7	0.80	76.7/75.4	11	0.93	80/90.6	14	0.99	100/93.5
Reiberger et al. [47] (n = 290)	N/S	N/S	N/S	7.2	0.690	73.3/77.4	9.6	0.737	86.9/82.9	12.1	0.904	84.8/86.8
Zarski et al. [38] (n = 382)	N/S	N/S	N/S	5.2	0.82	96.6/34.8	N/S	N/S	N/S	12.9	0.93	76.8/89.6
Lupsor et al. [10] (n = 1202)	5.3	0.879	84.99/73.21	7.4	0.889	80.32/83/97	9.1	0.941	88.8/88.3	13.2	0.970	93.75/93.31
Schwabl et al. [39] (n = 188)	N/S	N/S	N/S	7.2	0.852	N/S	N/S	N/S	N/S	14.5	0.852	N/S
Yoneda et al. [40] (n = 102)	5.5	0.838	84.6/71.4	7.8	0.906	77.9/90.0	10.4	0.952	88.1/91.1	11.3	0.907	90.0/83.8
Njei et al. [41] * (n = 756) [2]	N/S	N/S	N/S	4.5-7.2	N/S	97/64	N/S	N/S	N/S	11.8-14.6	N/S	90/87

* Meta-analysis, N/S = not specified. [1] The Ziol study investigated the effect of biopsy length on the diagnostic performance of LSM, providing AUROC values for small and large biopsies, respectively. [2] These studies evaluated the use of VCTE in HIV-HCV coinfection.

5. VCTE Performance for Cirrhosis Evaluation in HCV Patients

5.1. Diagnosis of Cirrhosis by VCTE

One of the greatest benefits of VCTE is the noninvasive diagnosis of cirrhosis. As previously implied, VCTE performs better at evaluating cirrhosis rather than evaluating fibrosis stages [48]. In the Talwalkar meta-analysis [49], the pooled estimates for sensitivity (Se) and specificity (Sp) for cirrhosis were 87% and 91%, respectively. However, the diagnostic threshold bias was an important cause of heterogeneity for pooled results. In 2007, Shaheen et al. [50] provided summary estimates for cirrhosis diagnosis with a Se and Sp of 85.6% and 93.2%, respectively, for LS exceeding 12.5 kPa and AUROC values of 0.95. In another meta-analysis by Stebbing et al. [51], the cutoff value of 15.08 kPa had 84.45% Se and 94.69% Sp. Tsochatzis et al. [52] evaluated the VCTE accuracy for cirrhosis prediction and reported a summary Se and Sp of 83% and 89%, respectively, at a diagnostic threshold of 15 ± 4 kPa. The latest meta-analysis by Ying et al. [53], demonstrated high Se (84%) and Sp (90%) of VCTE for assessing liver cirrhosis in HCV patients. These results suggest that VCTE performs better at ruling out rather than ruling in cirrhosis, with a negative predictive value greater than 90% [35,36,54].

In contrast, regarding US there are conflicting results. The US scoring system (USSS) proposed by Moon et al. [55] seemed to surpass VCTE for the diagnosis of overt cirrhosis, providing 89.2% Se and 69.4% Sp for USSS $\geq$ 6, while LSM $\geq$ 17.4 kPa had 77.6% Se and 61.4% Sp. Nevertheless, the Moon study had several limitations, considering that diverse etiologies included in the study provided lower AUROC values for LSM (0.729) than usual. Berzigotti et al. [56] found that among subjects with presumed cirrhosis, US is the better choice to diagnose cirrhosis, whereas VCTE is the preferred method to rule it out. Their combination increased the diagnostic accuracy, contrasting the results of the Zhang [13] and Wang [31] studies.

5.2. Screening for Portal Hypertension

Portal hypertension (PH) is a common clinical syndrome of CLD, hemodynamically defined by increased portal venous pressure and a hyperdynamic state [57,58]. In the early, compensated phases of cirrhosis, PH is mainly a result of intrahepatic resistance to portal blood flow due to morphological changes characterized by fibrosis [59]. Subsequently, as the disease progresses, the increase in portal pressure gradient leads to severe complications, consisting of portosystemic collaterals and varices [58]. In cirrhosis, hepatic venous pressure gradient (HVPG) is the standard PH assessment method, but it is invasive and expensive. A HVPG value greater than 10 mmHg represents the threshold for clinically significant portal hypertension (CSPH), a stage where PH complications might arise [58]. For these patients, compensated advanced CLD (cACLD) is an alternative term recommended by the Baveno VI criteria [60], mainly to indicate that the fibrosis progression is a continuum spectrum among asymptomatic patients.

Abdominal US is the primary imaging technique widely used for liver, spleen and portal venous system evaluation, since it can identify PH features, including splenomegaly, portal vein system dilatation, ascites, and portosystemic abdominal collaterals [61,62]. In particular, the incorporation of color and power Doppler enabled the appraisal of the left gastric vein (LGV) hemodynamics, the damping index, and the splenic Doppler pulsatility index [63–65]. Of note is the Lee study which reported higher diagnostic accuracy (AUC = 0.873) for splenic arterial resistive index compared to the accuracy of LSM (AUC = 0.745) in a cohort of 47 patients [66]. Nonetheless, existing data is insufficient to recommend Doppler measurements as a trustworthy substitute for HVPG [67].

VCTE proved to be an excellent diagnostic tool for identifying CSPH with a hierarchical summary receiver operating characteristic (HSROC) value of 0.93, reported in the Shi meta-analysis [59]. Table 2 summarizes the results of studies regarding the accuracy of LSM for the prediction of preclinical PH, CSPH, and severe PH (SPH). Carrion et al. [45] were the first to report the significant correlation between LSM and HVPG (Pearson coefficient, 0.84; $p < 0.001$) among patients with HCV recurrence after liver transplant. Over time, these results were confirmed by prospective and retrospective studies in patients with CLD [39,47,59,68–74]. Even though Schwabl et al. [39] concluded that the etiology was not a significant confounder for the correlation between LSM and HVPG, we decided to emphasize within our table the HCV positive subgroup for integrative purposes [75–78]. Overall, the AUROC ranged from 0.786 to 0.93 for a threshold of 8 to 8.74 kPa for preclinical PH, AUROC 0.74 to 0.99 for CSPH with the corresponding cutoff values ranging from 13.6 to 21.6 kPa, whilst SPH-related AUROC ranged from 0.721 to 0.92 with the associated cutoff values of 17.6 to 24.5 kPa. These results suggest that, even if the correlation between the two parameters does not allow accurate HVPG estimation, LS has great discriminative power for the presence of CSPH [27]. Recently, a multicenter study of 5648 patients proposed a novel set of cutoff values of <7 and >12 kPa for excluding and diagnosing compensated advanced liver disease. Lowering the dual threshold initially proposed by the Baveno VI consensus provided excellent Se (91%) for ruling out and Sp (92%) for ruling in cACLD, safely reducing the use of LB [60].

Table 2. Accuracy of LSM for the prediction of preclinical PH, CSPH, and SPH.

Grade of Portal Hypertension (PH)		Preclinical PH (≥5 mmHg)			Clinically Significant PH (≥10 mmHg)			Severe PH (≥12 mmHg)		
Study	Correlation Coefficient	Cutoff (kPa)	AUROC	Se/Sp (%)	Cutoff (kPa)	AUROC	Se/Sp (%)	Cutoff (kPa)	AUROC	Se/Sp (%)
Carrion et al. [45] (n = 129) [1,*]	0.84	8.74	0.93	90/81	N/S	0.94	N/S	N/S	N/S	N/S
Vizzutti et al. [75] (n = 61) *	0.81	N/S	N/S	N/S	13.6	0.99	97/92	17.6	0.92	94/81
Bureau et al. [76] (n = 150) *	0.858	N/S	N/S	N/S	21	0.971	89.9/93.2	N/S	N/S	N/S
Lemoine et al. [77] (n = 44) *	0.46	N/S	N/S	N/S	20.5	0.76 ± 0.07	63/70	N/S	N/S	N/S
Sanchez-C. et al. [78] (n = 38) [2,*]	0.46	N/S	N/S	N/S	14	0.80	92.86/50	23	0.80	82.61/66.67
Reiberger et al. [47] (n = 390)	0.838	8	0.830	95.3/71	18	0.892	80.3/86.9	20	0.899	84.4/86.5
Llop et al. [68] (n = 52) #	0.646	N/S	N/S	N/S	Rule out: 13.6 Rule in: 21	0.857	88/61 42/100	N/S	N/S	N/S
Schwabl et al. [39] (n = 188) #	0.846	N/S	N/S	N/S	16.1	0.957	94.8/86.9	N/S	N/S	N/S
Hong et al. [69] (n = 59) #	0.496	N/S	N/S	N/S	21.95	0.851	82.5/73.7	24.25	0.877	82.9/70.8
Augustin et al. [70] (n = 40) #	N/S	N/S	N/S	N/S	25	N/S	65/93	N/S	N/S	N/S
Kitson et al. [71] (n = 95) #	N/S	N/S	N/S	N/S	29.0	0.900	71.9/100	N/S	N/S	N/S
Zykus et al. [72] (n = 107) #	0.75	N/S	N/S	N/S	17.4	0.949	88/87.5	20.6	0.915	82.8/80
Procopet et al. [73] (n = 55) #	0.699	N/S	N/S	N/S	19.0 ± 13.3	0.926	N/S	N/S	N/S	N/S
Kumar et al. [74] (n = 326)	0.361	N/S	0.786	N/S	21.6	0.74	79/67	N/S	0.721	N/S

* Data displayed only for HCV infected patients. # mixed etiologies, mostly viral or alcoholic liver disease. [1] The Carrion study used the threshold ≥6 mmHg for the diagnosis of PH. [2] The Sanchez-Conde study evaluated correlation between LSM and HVPG in HIV-HCV coinfection.

5.3. Prognostic Significance of Liver Stiffness in Patients with HCV Cirrhosis

There is growing evidence to support the use of VCTE for risk stratification and prognosis [27] even in HCV cirrhosis. In a study of 1457 CHC patients, LS had stronger prognostic value for overall 5-year mortality compared to histological fibrosis staging [79]. In addition, LSM by VCTE has been validated as a prognostic quantitative marker for developing liver related complications, including esophageal varices (EV), variceal bleeding, hepatic decompensation, and HCC [79–82]. Recent data suggests that liver and spleen stiffness correlate considerably with HVPG among cirrhotic patients. In fact, spleen stiffness seems to be superior to LS for the prediction of PH and can even predict the late recurrence of HCC [83–85].

5.3.1. Prediction of Esophageal Varices (EV) and Variceal Hemorrhage by VCTE

In the past years, several studies sought to discover LS accuracy for predicting the presence and size of EV [35,70,75,76,78,86]. In general terms, the greater the LS value—the higher the risk of the patient to present EV and an increased degree of EV, respectively [80]. However, as illustrated by Kim et al. [80], the cutoff values vary widely among studies and VCTE accuracy is still inappropriate to replace HVPG or upper GI endoscopy in screening for EV presence or determining their grade [27,48]. However, it should be mentioned that there were no noninvasive methods that proved to be satisfactorily enough. Even if several studies [64] found that LGV hepatofugal flow substantially correlates with EV, Doppler parameters are still unsuited to be a surrogate for esophagogastroduodenoscopy or HVPG, mostly as a result of significant inter-observer variability [67]. The current reference standard for the detection and classification of EV remains the esophagogastroduodenoscopy procedure, in spite of being an invasive and expensive method [67]. Nonetheless, VCTE should be used as an initial noninvasive method for selecting patients in whom these invasive procedures are indicated [48]. Recent data suggests that the combination between LS, spleen dimensions, and platelet count significantly improves the diagnostic accuracy of EV [87]. In fact, according to the latest recommendations of the Baveno VI guidelines, upper GI endoscopy can be safely avoided among patients with a LS value of <20 kPa and a platelet count greater than 150 G/L [88].

5.3.2. The Prognostic Value of VCTE for HCC Development Prediction

In patients with CLD, abdominal US is the first-line investigation for the detection and characterization of FLLs and the main screening tool for HCC with 51–87% Se and 80–100% Sp [89–91]. The add-on of US contrast agents improved the overall diagnostic accuracy of conventional US, offering comparable performance to magnetic resonance imaging or computed tomography for FLLs evaluation [92]. However, even though US significantly improves HCC surveillance, it lacks prognostic power. Increasing evidence implies that noninvasive methods, such as VCTE, are not solely a substitute for LB, but also predictive for liver-related complications, in particular HCC development [48]. It is well known that the degree of fibrosis is by far the strongest risk factor for developing HCC in HCV patients [93]. A decade ago, Masuzaki et al. [94] were the first to describe the relationship between LS and HCC incidence in a Japanese cohort of 866 CHC patients. The hazard ratio (HR) for HCC incidence was 16.7, 20.9, 25.6 and 45.5 for LS values of 10.1–15.0 kPa, 15.2–20.0 kPa, 20.1–25.0 kPa, and >25.0 kPa, respectively ($p < 0.001$). Other longitudinal prospective studies evaluated the prognostic performance of VCTE for the prediction of HCC development in HCV patients, with cutoff values ranging between 12–50 kPa [81,95–99]. In addition, Feier et al. [96] surprisingly found that an IQR exceeding 39% of median LSM is another adequate indicator and essential predictor for the presence of HCC. Nonetheless, in order to confirm whether LS can actually foresee liver-related complications, these results require further validation through prospective studies conducted on large cohorts. In case these results are validated and standardized, VCTE might become an efficient method for the noninvasive screening of patients with CLD, with a possibility to classify them in different risk categories [16]. An interesting point to make is that the elastography parameter already provided effective risk prediction models, especially in patients with chronic hepatitis B infection [100–104]. However, existing literature does not provide any prediction model for HCV-related HCC risk.

Following the availability and efficacy of direct-acting antivirals (DAAs), several studies sought to elucidate their capability of reducing the HCC risk, and whether VCTE might become helpful in objectifying it. Some studies and one meta-analysis reported that the risk of de novo HCC development is similar or even diminished in the subgroup receiving antiviral treatment, compared to the general population [105–109]. However, the absolute risk in patients with cirrhosis remains high, regardless of therapy, which is why this subset of patients should be considered for ongoing HCC surveillance [110]. Elastography facilitates dynamic prediction of HCC, especially before and after the antiviral treatment. In terms of independent risk factors, increased baseline LS and other noninvasive markers of fibrosis, as well as a less than 30% decrease in LS, correlate significantly with the risk of developing HCC [111,112]. In addition, Ioannou et al. [113] developed and internally validated models that estimate the risk of HCC development after DAA therapy, improving HCC surveillance efforts. Nonetheless, their prediction models based on cirrhosis and sustained viral response (SVR) require further international endorsement. In a combined case report–literature review, Strazzulla et al. [114] described a particular case of recurrent HCC after successful DAA treatment in a HCV positive 53-year old patient that received liver transplantation. Although the literature is rather scarce, VCTE may also prove useful in evaluating liver disease progression towards HCC in HCV patients receiving liver transplantation [115].

6. VCTE Use for Longitudinal Monitoring in Detecting Fibrosis Regression and Predicting Complication Risk after Achieving Sustained Viral Response

As previously mentioned, the main endpoints in CHC patients are the detection of significant fibrosis ($\geq$F2) and cirrhosis (F4), which have been the definitive indication of antiviral therapy for a long time [27]. However, due to the large availability of highly efficient DAAs, it is expected that significant fibrosis will no longer be a critical decision-making endpoint among these subjects [48].

VCTE, serving as a novel noninvasive method for fibrosis assessment, facilitates the longitudinal evaluation of HCV patients, before and after antiviral treatment. However, fibrosis and PH regression in patients with treated HCV-related cirrhosis is still a debatable subject [116]. Several studies explored the dynamics of LS in patients receiving antiviral therapy (interferon based/interferon-free therapies), concluding that the LS values decreased significantly in those with SVR [111,117–129]. Most of these studies showed better improvement of LS among patients with higher pre-treatment fibrosis stages [111,117–122,129]. However, Persico et al. [124] found that EV of any size anticipated a lack of LS improvement. A study by Chan et al. [125] reported that a baseline elevated ALT was independently associated with a reduction of LS beyond 30%. As assumed by some researchers, this might come as a result of substantial decrease of liver inflammation, rather than fibrosis regression, at the end of the antiviral therapy [116,128,130–132]. Nonetheless, several reports showed that liver fibrosis reverses in approximately one third to nearly half of CHC patients [133]. Of note is the D'Ambrosio study, which found significant cirrhosis regression by LB in 61% of individuals with HCV-related cirrhosis [134].

7. Controlled Attenuation Parameter (CAP) for the Noninvasive Evaluation of Steatosis in HCV-Infected Patients

Besides fibrosis, steatosis is another common histological feature in HCV patients, especially those infected with genotype 3 [135]. Viral contamination is an independent risk factor for fat accumulation in HCV patients, along with obesity, type II diabetes mellitus, and alcohol consumption. Steatosis was found to be 1.5–2.5 times more prevalent among these subjects than in the general population [136]. In fact, several studies reported that steatosis might increase fibrosis progression and the risk of HCC development while lowering the response rate to antiviral treatment [137–140]. Therefore, steatosis assessment in HCV positive individuals is of great importance.

At present, abdominal conventional US is the most readily available, simple and cost-effective technique for steatosis appraisal in clinical setting [141]. A 2011 meta-analysis by Hernaez et al. [142] confirmed that B-mode US is a reliable method for steatosis assessment in comparison to liver biopsy. Among 4720 patients, liver US provided 84.8% Se (95% CI: 79.5–88.9), 93.6% Sp (95% CI: 87.2–97.0) and AUROC of 0.93 (95% CI: 0.91–0.95) for moderate to severe steatosis detection. However, its sensitivity lowers when less than 30% of the hepatocytes are affected. Besides, it remains a subjective method, resulting in high variability and low reproducibility [141]. The introduction of the hepatorenal Index (HRI) sought to overcome this drawback, providing excellent diagnostic precision for the diagnosis of steatosis (>5%) with AUROC of 0.99, 100% Se and 91% Sp [143]. Novel quantitative US parameters from radiofrequency data analysis show promising results, surpassing the HRI [144].

Furthermore, numerous studies investigated the use of the novel CAP for steatosis evaluation, as a substitute for the invasive LB [145–147]. Several meta-analyses offered consistent results, with AUROC values ranging from 0.81–0.96 for the detection of mild steatosis ($\geq$S1), 0.82–0.90 for moderate steatosis ($\geq$S2), and 0.70–0.97 for severe steatosis ($\geq$S3) [148–150]. In 2017, an individual patients' data meta-analysis, involving 2735 CLD subjects, provided cutoff values of 148 dB/m, 286 dB/m and 280 dB/m for the presence of mild, moderate, and severe steatosis, respectively, using the M probe [23]. However, novel data suggests that optimal cutoff values vary significantly by both probes across different etiologies. Regarding HCV patients, the latest comprehensive meta-analysis could not analyze in great detail this pathology, due to the small cohort and low prevalence of high-grade steatosis [25]. Therefore, additional data concerning this etiology is still needed. Regarding performance, the Moret study found that the hepatorenal B-mode ratio and CAP have comparable power for the diagnosis of steatosis ($\geq$S1), but both lack the ability to discern between moderate to severe steatosis [151].

Moreover, studies show conflicting results with the use of CAP for steatosis evaluation in the context of the new DAA therapy. On one hand, Rout et al. [152] and Ogasawara et al. [153] reported that the CAP score tends to increase in patients treated with DAAs, but these studies could not find an explanation for this phenomenon. On the other hand, two other papers found that DAAs significantly lower hepatic steatosis in chronic HCV patients with fatty liver, while the Sung study noted significant steatosis reduction only in patients with moderate fatty infiltration (S0-S1) at baseline evaluation [154–156]. Nevertheless, CAP remains a powerful add-on in the management of HCV patients.

8. Advantages and Limitations of VCTE

Although VCTE is increasingly used in daily practice as a noninvasive and efficient method of assessing liver stiffness, it has several limitations. Technically, VCTE cannot be performed in patients with ascites because the elastic waves are not able to penetrate the fluids. Moreover, VCTE is limited by the narrow intercostal space and some obese patients present a challenge in the VCTE examination. In obese patients, the XL probe is required in order to reduce the failure rate [10,26,48,157]. Furthermore, in a multivariate analysis by Castera et al. [20], the only factor associated with failure was obesity (body mass index > 28 kg/m^2, $p < 0.001$) and VCTE was not successful in 20% of cases. Other factors, such as abdominal wall edema or congestion, can alter the measurements and increase the stiffness, independently of fibrosis.

From another point of view, the main limitations are the need for a dedicated device, which is not always available, and the fact that it is not possible to choose a region of interest for the measurements. Individual factors related to the patient's condition, such as acute hepatitis, increased transaminases, extrahepatic cholestasis, congestion, and food or excessive alcohol intake could increase liver stiffness, resulting in false positive results [27].

9. Concluding Remarks

In the current paper, we have critically reviewed VCTE performance in the assessment of HCV patients, highlighting the advantages of this ultrasound elastographic technique in comparison to conventional US. Besides staging liver fibrosis, the high specificity and negative predictive value of VCTE suggest that it performs better at ruling out cirrhosis rather than diagnosing it. Furthermore, the high hierarchical summary receiver operating characteristic of VCTE in diagnosing CSPH proved the efficacy of this ultrasound elastography method in identifying CSPH. The current range of LS cutoff values for predicting the presence and size of the esophageal varices are wide and standardized values are not available. However, a general rule is that 'the greater the stiffness, the higher the possibility of esophageal varices and their diameter'. Whilst existing literature suggests that VCTE can be used for HCC risk prediction in other hepatopathies, there are currently no indications for risk prediction in HCV. This would be an important application, as VCTE already allows patient stratification through risk assessment in some instances. One of its upsides that opened a new era in HCV management is that it can be repeated every time it is deemed necessary—before antiviral therapy, in monitoring fibrosis regression after HCV eradication. As such, the advantages of VCTE significantly outweigh those of other surveillance methods.

Our opinion is that HCV patients can greatly benefit from VCTE due to its numerous qualities—rapid, noninvasive, repeatable for longitudinal evaluation and the cost-effectiveness. We propose that further studies should focus on establishing standardized cutoff values of LS for predicting the presence and size of esophageal varices, as well as investigating the potential for predicting HCC risk in HCV patients, which is considered to be of great importance in current clinical practice.

Author Contributions: Conceptualization—all authors; writing—M.F., T.S., G.R.T., A.T.; writing—review—all authors; critically revising—M.L.-P., M.F.; project administration—M.L.-P. All authors have read and agreed to the published version of the manuscript.

Funding: This research received no external funding.

Conflicts of Interest: The authors declare no conflict of interest.

References

1. Ahmad, J. Hepatitis C. *BMJ* **2017**, *358*, j2861. [CrossRef]
2. Jafri, S.M.; Gordon, S.C. Epidemiology of Hepatitis C. *Clin. Liver Dis. Hoboken* **2018**, *12*, 140–142. [CrossRef]
3. Li, H.C.; Lo, S.Y. Hepatitis C virus: Virology, diagnosis and treatment. *World J. Hepatol.* **2015**, *7*, 1377–1389. [CrossRef]
4. Morozov, V.A.; Lagaye, S. Hepatitis C virus: Morphogenesis, infection and therapy. *World J. Hepatol.* **2018**, *10*, 186–212. [CrossRef]
5. Kennedy, P.; Wagner, M.; Castera, L.; Hong, C.W.; Johnson, C.L.; Sirlin, C.B.; Taouli, B. Quantitative Elastography Methods in Liver Disease: Current Evidence and Future Directions. *Radiology* **2018**, *286*, 738–763. [CrossRef]
6. Sirinawasatien, A.; Techasirioangkun, T. The Prevalence and Determinants of Hepatic Steatosis Assessed by Controlled Attenuation Parameter in Thai Chronic Hepatitis C Patients. *Gastroenterol. Res. Pract.* **2020**, *2020*, 8814135. [CrossRef] [PubMed]
7. Lupsor, M.; Badea, R.; Nedevschi, S.; Mitrea, D.; Florea, M. Ultrasonography Contribution to Hepatic Steatosis Quantification. Possibilities of Improving this Method through Computerized Analysis of Ultrasonic Image. In Proceedings of the 2006 IEEE International Conference on Automation, Quality and Testing, Robotics, Cluj-Napoca, Romania, 25–28 May 2006; pp. 478–483.
8. Trivedi, H.D.; Lin, S.C.; Lau, D.T.Y. Noninvasive Assessment of Fibrosis Regression in Hepatitis C Virus Sustained Virologic Responders. *Gastroenterol. Hepatol. N. Y.* **2017**, *13*, 587–595. [PubMed]
9. Seeff, L.B.; Everson, G.T.; Morgan, T.R.; Curto, T.M.; Lee, W.M.; Ghany, M.G.; Shiffman, M.L.; Fontana, R.J.; Di Bisceglie, A.M.; Bonkovsky, H.L.; et al. Complication rate of percutaneous liver biopsies among persons with advanced chronic liver disease in the HALT-C trial. *Clin. Gastroenterol. Hepatol.* **2010**, *8*, 877–883. [CrossRef]
10. Lupsor Platon, M.; Stefanescu, H.; Feier, D.; Maniu, A.; Badea, R. Performance of unidimensional transient elastography in staging chronic hepatitis C. Results from a cohort of 1202 biopsied patients from one single center. *J. Gastrointestin Liver Dis.* **2013**, *22*, 157–166. [PubMed]
11. Patel, K.; Sebastiani, G. Limitations of non-invasive tests for assessment of liver fibrosis. *JHEP Rep.* **2020**, *2*, 100067. [CrossRef]
12. Barr, R.G. Ultrasound of Diffuse Liver Disease Including Elastography. *Radiol. Clin. N. Am.* **2019**, *57*, 549–562. [CrossRef]
13. Zhang, G.L.; Zhao, Q.Y.; Lin, C.S.; Hu, Z.X.; Zhang, T.; Gao, Z.L. Transient Elastography and Ultrasonography: Optimal Evaluation of Liver Fibrosis and Cirrhosis in Patients with Chronic Hepatitis B Concurrent with Nonalcoholic Fatty Liver Disease. *Biomed. Res. Int.* **2019**, *2019*, 3951574. [CrossRef] [PubMed]

14. Singh, T.; Allende, D.S.; McCullough, A.J. Assessing liver fibrosis without biopsy in patients with HCV or NAFLD. *Cleve Clin. J. Med.* **2019**, *86*, 179–186. [CrossRef] [PubMed]
15. Lupsor-Platon, M.; Serban, T.; Silion, A.I.; Tirpe, A.; Florea, M. Hepatocellular Carcinoma and Non-Alcoholic Fatty Liver Disease: A Step Forward for Better Evaluation Using Ultrasound Elastography. *Cancers* **2020**, *12*, 2778. [CrossRef]
16. Lupsor Platon, M. Noninvasive Assessment of Diffuse Liver Diseases Using Vibration-Controlled Transient Elastography (VCTE). In *Ultrasound Elastography*; IntechOpen: London, UK, 2019. [CrossRef]
17. Arena, U.; Lupsor Platon, M.; Stasi, C.; Moscarella, S.; Assarat, A.; Bedogni, G.; Piazzolla, V.; Badea, R.; Laffi, G.; Marra, F.; et al. Liver stiffness is influenced by a standardized meal in patients with chronic hepatitis C virus at different stages of fibrotic evolution. *Hepatology* **2013**, *58*, 65–72. [CrossRef]
18. Tapper, E.B.; Castera, L.; Afdhal, N.H. FibroScan (vibration-controlled transient elastography): Where does it stand in the United States practice. *Clin. Gastroenterol. Hepatol.* **2015**, *13*, 27–36. [CrossRef]
19. Bonder, A.; Afdhal, N. Utilization of FibroScan in clinical practice. *Curr. Gastroenterol. Rep.* **2014**, *16*, 372. [CrossRef]
20. Castera, L.; Foucher, J.; Bernard, P.H.; Carvalho, F.; Allaix, D.; Merrouche, W.; Couzigou, P.; de Ledinghen, V. Pitfalls of liver stiffness measurement: A 5-year prospective study of 13,369 examinations. *Hepatology* **2010**, *51*, 828–835. [CrossRef]
21. Pang, J.X.; Pradhan, F.; Zimmer, S.; Niu, S.; Crotty, P.; Tracey, J.; Schneider, C.; Heitman, S.J.; Kaplan, G.G.; Swain, M.G.; et al. The feasibility and reliability of transient elastography using Fibroscan(R): A practice audit of 2335 examinations. *Can. J. Gastroenterol. Hepatol.* **2014**, *28*, 143–149. [CrossRef]
22. Tapper, E.B.; Afdhal, N.H. Vibration-controlled transient elastography: A practical approach to the noninvasive assessment of liver fibrosis. *Curr. Opin. Gastroenterol.* **2015**, *31*, 192–198. [CrossRef]
23. Karlas, T.; Petroff, D.; Sasso, M.; Fan, J.G.; Mi, Y.Q.; de Ledinghen, V.; Kumar, M.; Lupsor-Platon, M.; Han, K.H.; Cardoso, A.C.; et al. Individual patient data meta-analysis of controlled attenuation parameter (CAP) technology for assessing steatosis. *J. Hepatol.* **2017**, *66*, 1022–1030. [CrossRef]
24. Chon, Y.E.; Jung, K.S.; Kim, K.J.; Joo, D.J.; Kim, B.K.; Park, J.Y.; Kim, D.Y.; Ahn, S.H.; Han, K.H.; Kim, S.U. Normal controlled attenuation parameter values: A prospective study of healthy subjects undergoing health checkups and liver donors in Korea. *Dig. Dis. Sci.* **2015**, *60*, 234–242. [CrossRef] [PubMed]
25. Petroff, D.; Blank, V.; Newsome, P.N.; Shalimar, V.C.S.; Thiele, M.; de Lédinghen, V.; Baumeler, S.; Chan, W.K.; Perlemuter, G. Assessment of hepatic steatosis by controlled attenuation parameter using the M and XL probes: An individual patient data meta-analysis. *Lancet Gastroenterol. Hepatol.* **2021**. [CrossRef]
26. Lupsor, M.; Badea, R.; Stefanescu, H.; Grigorescu, M.; Sparchez, Z.; Serban, A.; Branda, H.; Iancu, S.; Maniu, A. Analysis of histopathological changes that influence liver stiffness in chronic hepatitis C. Results from a cohort of 324 patients. *J. Gastrointestin Liver Dis.* **2008**, *17*, 155–163.
27. Dietrich, C.F.; Bamber, J.; Berzigotti, A.; Bota, S.; Cantisani, V.; Castera, L.; Cosgrove, D.; Ferraioli, G.; Friedrich-Rust, M.; Gilja, O.H.; et al. EFSUMB Guidelines and Recommendations on the Clinical Use of Liver Ultrasound Elastography, Update 2017 (Long Version). *Ultraschall Med.* **2017**, *38*, e16–e47. [CrossRef]
28. Adolf, S.; Millonig, G.; Friedrich, S.; Seitz, H.K.; Mueller, S. Valsalva and orthostatic maneuvers increase liver stiffness (Fibroscan®) in healthy volunteers. *Z. Gastroenterol.* **2010**, *48*. [CrossRef]
29. Coco, B.; Oliveri, F.; Maina, A.M.; Ciccorossi, P.; Sacco, R.; Colombatto, P.; Bonino, F.; Brunetto, M.R. Transient elastography: A new surrogate marker of liver fibrosis influenced by major changes of transaminases. *J. Viral. Hepat.* **2007**, *14*, 360–369. [CrossRef]
30. Bota, S.; Sporea, I.; Peck-Radosavljevic, M.; Sirli, R.; Tanaka, H.; Iijima, H.; Saito, H.; Ebinuma, H.; Lupsor, M.; Badea, R.; et al. The influence of aminotransferase levels on liver stiffness assessed by Acoustic Radiation Force Impulse Elastography: A retrospective multicentre study. *Dig. Liver Dis.* **2013**, *45*, 762–768. [CrossRef]
31. Wang, J.H.; Changchien, C.S.; Hung, C.H.; Eng, H.L.; Tung, W.C.; Kee, K.M.; Chen, C.H.; Hu, T.H.; Lee, C.M.; Lu, S.N. FibroScan and ultrasonography in the prediction of hepatic fibrosis in patients with chronic viral hepatitis. *J. Gastroenterol.* **2009**, *44*, 439–446. [CrossRef]
32. Brener, S. Transient Elastography for Assessment of Liver Fibrosis and Steatosis: An Evidence-Based Analysis. *Ont. Health Technol. Assess. Ser.* **2015**, *15*, 1–45. [PubMed]
33. Sandrin, L.; Fourquet, B.; Hasquenoph, J.M.; Yon, S.; Fournier, C.; Mal, F.; Christidis, C.; Ziol, M.; Poulet, B.; Kazemi, F.; et al. Transient elastography: A new noninvasive method for assessment of hepatic fibrosis. *Ultrasound Med. Biol.* **2003**, *29*, 1705–1713. [CrossRef]
34. Ziol, M.; Handra-Luca, A.; Kettaneh, A.; Christidis, C.; Mal, F.; Kazemi, F.; de Ledinghen, V.; Marcellin, P.; Dhumeaux, D.; Trinchet, J.C.; et al. Noninvasive assessment of liver fibrosis by measurement of stiffness in patients with chronic hepatitis C. *Hepatology* **2005**, *41*, 48–54. [CrossRef]
35. Castera, L.; Vergniol, J.; Foucher, J.; Le Bail, B.; Chanteloup, E.; Haaser, M.; Darriet, M.; Couzigou, P.; De Ledinghen, V. Prospective comparison of transient elastography, Fibrotest, APRI, and liver biopsy for the assessment of fibrosis in chronic hepatitis C. *Gastroenterology* **2005**, *128*, 343–350. [CrossRef]
36. De Ledinghen, V.; Douvin, C.; Kettaneh, A.; Ziol, M.; Roulot, D.; Marcellin, P.; Dhumeaux, D.; Beaugrand, M. Diagnosis of hepatic fibrosis and cirrhosis by transient elastography in HIV/hepatitis C virus-coinfected patients. *J. Acquir. Immune Defic. Syndr.* **2006**, *41*, 175–179. [CrossRef]

37. Arena, U.; Vizzutti, F.; Abraldes, J.G.; Corti, G.; Stasi, C.; Moscarella, S.; Milani, S.; Lorefice, E.; Petrarca, A.; Romanelli, R.G.; et al. Reliability of transient elastography for the diagnosis of advanced fibrosis in chronic hepatitis C. *Gut* **2008**, *57*, 1288–1293. [CrossRef] [PubMed]
38. Zarski, J.P.; Sturm, N.; Guechot, J.; Paris, A.; Zafrani, E.S.; Asselah, T.; Boisson, R.C.; Bosson, J.L.; Guyader, D.; Renversez, J.C.; et al. Comparison of nine blood tests and transient elastography for liver fibrosis in chronic hepatitis C: The ANRS HCEP-23 study. *J. Hepatol.* **2012**, *56*, 55–62. [CrossRef] [PubMed]
39. Schwabl, P.; Bota, S.; Salzl, P.; Mandorfer, M.; Payer, B.A.; Ferlitsch, A.; Stift, J.; Wrba, F.; Trauner, M.; Peck-Radosavljevic, M.; et al. New reliability criteria for transient elastography increase the number of accurate measurements for screening of cirrhosis and portal hypertension. *Liver Int.* **2015**, *35*, 381–390. [CrossRef] [PubMed]
40. Yoneda, M.; Thomas, E.; Sclair, S.N.; Grant, T.T.; Schiff, E.R. Supersonic Shear Imaging and Transient Elastography With the XL Probe Accurately Detect Fibrosis in Overweight or Obese Patients With Chronic Liver Disease. *Clin. Gastroenterol. Hepatol.* **2015**, *13*, 1502–1509.e5. [CrossRef] [PubMed]
41. Njei, B.; McCarty, T.R.; Luk, J.; Ewelukwa, O.; Ditah, I.; Lim, J.K. Use of transient elastography in patients with HIV-HCV coinfection: A systematic review and meta-analysis. *J. Gastroenterol. Hepatol.* **2016**, *31*, 1684–1693. [CrossRef]
42. Sanchez-Conde, M.; Montes-Ramirez, M.L.; Miralles, P.; Alvarez, J.M.; Bellon, J.M.; Ramirez, M.; Arribas, J.R.; Gutierrez, I.; Lopez, J.C.; Cosin, J.; et al. Comparison of transient elastography and liver biopsy for the assessment of liver fibrosis in HIV/hepatitis C virus-coinfected patients and correlation with noninvasive serum markers. *J. Viral. Hepat.* **2010**, *17*, 280–286. [CrossRef]
43. Nitta, Y.; Kawabe, N.; Hashimoto, S.; Harata, M.; Komura, N.; Kobayashi, K.; Arima, Y.; Shimazaki, H.; Nakano, T.; Murao, M.; et al. Liver stiffness measured by transient elastography correlates with fibrosis area in liver biopsy in patients with chronic hepatitis C. *Hepatol. Res.* **2009**, *39*, 675–684. [CrossRef]
44. Poynard, T.; Halfon, P.; Castera, L.; Munteanu, M.; Imbert-Bismut, F.; Ratziu, V.; Benhamou, Y.; Bourliere, M.; de Ledinghen, V.; FibroPaca, G. Standardization of ROC curve areas for diagnostic evaluation of liver fibrosis markers based on prevalences of fibrosis stages. *Clin. Chem.* **2007**, *53*, 1615–1622. [CrossRef]
45. Carrion, J.A.; Navasa, M.; Bosch, J.; Bruguera, M.; Gilabert, R.; Forns, X. Transient elastography for diagnosis of advanced fibrosis and portal hypertension in patients with hepatitis C recurrence after liver transplantation. *Liver Transpl.* **2006**, *12*, 1791–1798. [CrossRef] [PubMed]
46. Sporea, I.; Sirli, R.; Deleanu, A.; Tudora, A.; Curescu, M.; Cornianu, M.; Lazar, D. Comparison of the liver stiffness measurement by transient elastography with the liver biopsy. *World J. Gastroenterol.* **2008**, *14*, 6513–6517. [CrossRef]
47. Reiberger, T.; Ferlitsch, A.; Payer, B.A.; Pinter, M.; Schwabl, P.; Stift, J.; Trauner, M.; Peck-Radosavljevic, M. Noninvasive screening for liver fibrosis and portal hypertension by transient elastography—A large single center experience. *Wien. Klin. Wochenschr.* **2012**, *124*, 395–402. [CrossRef]
48. European Association for Study of Liver; Asociacion Latinoamericana para el Estudio del Higado. EASL-ALEH Clinical Practice Guidelines: Non-invasive tests for evaluation of liver disease severity and prognosis. *J. Hepatol.* **2015**, *63*, 237–264. [CrossRef]
49. Talwalkar, J.A.; Kurtz, D.M.; Schoenleber, S.J.; West, C.P.; Montori, V.M. Ultrasound-based transient elastography for the detection of hepatic fibrosis: Systematic review and meta-analysis. *Clin. Gastroenterol. Hepatol.* **2007**, *5*, 1214–1220. [CrossRef]
50. Shaheen, A.A.; Wan, A.F.; Myers, R.P. FibroTest and FibroScan for the prediction of hepatitis C-related fibrosis: A systematic review of diagnostic test accuracy. *Am. J. Gastroenterol.* **2007**, *102*, 2589–2600. [CrossRef]
51. Stebbing, J.; Farouk, L.; Panos, G.; Anderson, M.; Jiao, L.R.; Mandalia, S.; Bower, M.; Gazzard, B.; Nelson, M. A meta-analysis of transient elastography for the detection of hepatic fibrosis. *J. Clin. Gastroenterol.* **2010**, *44*, 214–219. [CrossRef]
52. Tsochatzis, E.A.; Gurusamy, K.S.; Ntaoula, S.; Cholongitas, E.; Davidson, B.R.; Burroughs, A.K. Elastography for the diagnosis of severity of fibrosis in chronic liver disease: A meta-analysis of diagnostic accuracy. *J. Hepatol.* **2011**, *54*, 650–659. [CrossRef]
53. Ying, H.Y.; Lu, L.G.; Jing, D.D.; Ni, X.S. Accuracy of transient elastography in the assessment of chronic hepatitis C-related liver cirrhosis. *Clin. Investig. Med.* **2016**, *39*, E150–E160. [CrossRef]
54. Colletta, C.; Smirne, C.; Fabris, C.; Toniutto, P.; Rapetti, R.; Minisini, R.; Pirisi, M. Value of two noninvasive methods to detect progression of fibrosis among HCV carriers with normal aminotransferases. *Hepatology* **2005**, *42*, 838–845. [CrossRef]
55. Moon, K.M.; Kim, G.; Baik, S.K.; Choi, E.; Kim, M.Y.; Kim, H.A.; Cho, M.Y.; Shin, S.Y.; Kim, J.M.; Park, H.J.; et al. Ultrasonographic scoring system score versus liver stiffness measurement in prediction of cirrhosis. *Clin. Mol. Hepatol.* **2013**, *19*, 389–398. [CrossRef] [PubMed]
56. Berzigotti, A.; Abraldes, J.G.; Tandon, P.; Erice, E.; Gilabert, R.; Garcia-Pagan, J.C.; Bosch, J. Ultrasonographic evaluation of liver surface and transient elastography in clinically doubtful cirrhosis. *J. Hepatol.* **2010**, *52*, 846–853. [CrossRef]
57. Gunarathne, L.S.; Rajapaksha, H.; Shackel, N.; Angus, P.W.; Herath, C.B. Cirrhotic portal hypertension: From pathophysiology to novel therapeutics. *World J. Gastroenterol.* **2020**, *26*, 6111–6140. [CrossRef]
58. Bosch, J.; Abraldes, J.G.; Berzigotti, A.; Garcia-Pagan, J.C. The clinical use of HVPG measurements in chronic liver disease. *Nat. Rev. Gastroenterol. Hepatol.* **2009**, *6*, 573–582. [CrossRef]
59. Shi, K.Q.; Fan, Y.C.; Pan, Z.Z.; Lin, X.F.; Liu, W.Y.; Chen, Y.P.; Zheng, M.H. Transient elastography: A meta-analysis of diagnostic accuracy in evaluation of portal hypertension in chronic liver disease. *Liver Int.* **2013**, *33*, 62–71. [CrossRef]
60. Papatheodoridi, M.; Hiriart, J.B.; Lupsor-Platon, M.; Bronte, F.; Boursier, J.; Elshaarawy, O.; Marra, F.; Thiele, M.; Markakis, G.; Payance, A.; et al. Refining the Baveno VI elastography criteria for the definition of compensated advanced chronic liver disease. *J. Hepatol.* **2021**, *74*, 1109–1116. [CrossRef]

61. Berzigotti, A.; Piscaglia, F.; Education, E.; Professional Standards, C. Ultrasound in portal hypertension—Part 2—And EFSUMB recommendations for the performance and reporting of ultrasound examinations in portal hypertension. *Ultraschall Med.* **2012**, *33*, 8–32; quiz 30–31. [CrossRef] [PubMed]
62. Berzigotti, A.; Piscaglia, F. Ultrasound in portal hypertension—Part 1. *Ultraschall Med.* **2011**, *32*, 548–568; quiz 569–571. [CrossRef]
63. Kim, M.Y.; Baik, S.K.; Park, D.H.; Lim, D.W.; Kim, J.W.; Kim, H.S.; Kwon, S.O.; Kim, Y.J.; Chang, S.J.; Lee, S.S. Damping index of Doppler hepatic vein waveform to assess the severity of portal hypertension and response to propranolol in liver cirrhosis: A prospective nonrandomized study. *Liver Int.* **2007**, *27*, 1103–1110. [CrossRef] [PubMed]
64. Cannella, R.; Giambelluca, D.; Pellegrinelli, A.; Cabassa, P. Color Doppler Ultrasound in Portal Hypertension: A Closer Look at Left Gastric Vein Hemodynamics. *J. Ultrasound Med.* **2021**, *40*, 7–14. [CrossRef]
65. Bolognesi, M.; Sacerdoti, D.; Merkel, C.; Bombonato, G.; Gatta, A. Noninvasive grading of the severity of portal hypertension in cirrhotic patients by echo-color-Doppler. *Ultrasound Med. Biol.* **2001**, *27*, 901–907. [CrossRef]
66. Lee, C.M.; Jeong, W.K.; Lim, S.; Kim, Y.; Kim, J.; Kim, T.Y.; Sohn, J.H. Diagnosis of Clinically Significant Portal Hypertension in Patients with Cirrhosis: Splenic Arterial Resistive Index versus Liver Stiffness Measurement. *Ultrasound Med. Biol.* **2016**, *42*, 1312–1320. [CrossRef]
67. Qi, X.; Berzigotti, A.; Cardenas, A.; Sarin, S.K. Emerging non-invasive approaches for diagnosis and monitoring of portal hypertension. *Lancet Gastroenterol. Hepatol.* **2018**, *3*, 708–719. [CrossRef]
68. Llop, E.; Berzigotti, A.; Reig, M.; Erice, E.; Reverter, E.; Seijo, S.; Abraldes, J.G.; Bruix, J.; Bosch, J.; Garcia-Pagan, J.C. Assessment of portal hypertension by transient elastography in patients with compensated cirrhosis and potentially resectable liver tumors. *J. Hepatol.* **2012**, *56*, 103–108. [CrossRef]
69. Hong, W.K.; Kim, M.Y.; Baik, S.K.; Shin, S.Y.; Kim, J.M.; Kang, Y.S.; Lim, Y.L.; Kim, Y.J.; Cho, Y.Z.; Hwang, H.W.; et al. The usefulness of non-invasive liver stiffness measurements in predicting clinically significant portal hypertension in cirrhotic patients: Korean data. *Clin. Mol. Hepatol.* **2013**, *19*, 370–375. [CrossRef]
70. Augustin, S.; Millan, L.; Gonzalez, A.; Martell, M.; Gelabert, A.; Segarra, A.; Serres, X.; Esteban, R.; Genesca, J. Detection of early portal hypertension with routine data and liver stiffness in patients with asymptomatic liver disease: A prospective study. *J. Hepatol.* **2014**, *60*, 561–569. [CrossRef]
71. Kitson, M.T.; Roberts, S.K.; Colman, J.C.; Paul, E.; Button, P.; Kemp, W. Liver stiffness and the prediction of clinically significant portal hypertension and portal hypertensive complications. *Scand. J. Gastroenterol.* **2015**, *50*, 462–469. [CrossRef]
72. Zykus, R.; Jonaitis, L.; Petrenkiene, V.; Pranculis, A.; Kupcinskas, L. Liver and spleen transient elastography predicts portal hypertension in patients with chronic liver disease: A prospective cohort study. *BMC Gastroenterol.* **2015**, *15*, 183. [CrossRef] [PubMed]
73. Procopet, B.; Berzigotti, A.; Abraldes, J.G.; Turon, F.; Hernandez-Gea, V.; Garcia-Pagan, J.C.; Bosch, J. Real-time shear-wave elastography: Applicability, reliability and accuracy for clinically significant portal hypertension. *J. Hepatol.* **2015**, *62*, 1068–1075. [CrossRef]
74. Kumar, A.; Khan, N.M.; Anikhindi, S.A.; Sharma, P.; Bansal, N.; Singla, V.; Arora, A. Correlation of transient elastography with hepatic venous pressure gradient in patients with cirrhotic portal hypertension: A study of 326 patients from India. *World J. Gastroenterol.* **2017**, *23*, 687–696. [CrossRef] [PubMed]
75. Vizzutti, F.; Arena, U.; Romanelli, R.G.; Rega, L.; Foschi, M.; Colagrande, S.; Petrarca, A.; Moscarella, S.; Belli, G.; Zignego, A.L.; et al. Liver stiffness measurement predicts severe portal hypertension in patients with HCV-related cirrhosis. *Hepatology* **2007**, *45*, 1290–1297. [CrossRef]
76. Bureau, C.; Metivier, S.; Peron, J.M.; Selves, J.; Robic, M.A.; Gourraud, P.A.; Rouquet, O.; Dupuis, E.; Alric, L.; Vinel, J.P. Transient elastography accurately predicts presence of significant portal hypertension in patients with chronic liver disease. *Aliment. Pharm.* **2008**, *27*, 1261–1268. [CrossRef] [PubMed]
77. Lemoine, M.; Katsahian, S.; Ziol, M.; Nahon, P.; Ganne-Carrie, N.; Kazemi, F.; Grando-Lemaire, V.; Trinchet, J.C.; Beaugrand, M. Liver stiffness measurement as a predictive tool of clinically significant portal hypertension in patients with compensated hepatitis C virus or alcohol-related cirrhosis. *Aliment. Pharm.* **2008**, *28*, 1102–1110. [CrossRef]
78. Sanchez-Conde, M.; Miralles, P.; Bellon, J.M.; Rincon, D.; Ramirez, M.; Gutierrez, I.; Ripoll, C.; Lopez, J.C.; Cosin, J.; Clemente, G.; et al. Use of transient elastography (FibroScan(R)) for the noninvasive assessment of portal hypertension in HIV/HCV-coinfected patients. *J. Viral Hepat.* **2011**, *18*, 685–691. [CrossRef]
79. Vergniol, J.; Foucher, J.; Terrebonne, E.; Bernard, P.H.; le Bail, B.; Merrouche, W.; Couzigou, P.; de Ledinghen, V. Noninvasive tests for fibrosis and liver stiffness predict 5-year outcomes of patients with chronic hepatitis C. *Gastroenterology* **2011**, *140*, 1970–1979.e3. [CrossRef] [PubMed]
80. Kim, B.K.; Fung, J.; Yuen, M.F.; Kim, S.U. Clinical application of liver stiffness measurement using transient elastography in chronic liver disease from longitudinal perspectives. *World J. Gastroenterol.* **2013**, *19*, 1890–1900. [CrossRef] [PubMed]
81. Poynard, T.; Vergniol, J.; Ngo, Y.; Foucher, J.; Munteanu, M.; Merrouche, W.; Colombo, M.; Thibault, V.; Schiff, E.; Brass, C.A.; et al. Staging chronic hepatitis C in seven categories using fibrosis biomarker (FibroTest) and transient elastography (FibroScan(R)). *J. Hepatol.* **2014**, *60*, 706–714. [CrossRef] [PubMed]
82. Robic, M.A.; Procopet, B.; Metivier, S.; Peron, J.M.; Selves, J.; Vinel, J.P.; Bureau, C. Liver stiffness accurately predicts portal hypertension related complications in patients with chronic liver disease: A prospective study. *J. Hepatol.* **2011**, *55*, 1017–1024. [CrossRef]

83. Tseng, Y.; Li, F.; Wang, J.; Chen, S.; Jiang, W.; Shen, X.; Wu, S. Spleen and liver stiffness for noninvasive assessment of portal hypertension in cirrhotic patients with large esophageal varices. *J. Clin. Ultrasound* **2018**, *46*, 442–449. [CrossRef]
84. Marasco, G.; Colecchia, A.; Colli, A.; Ravaioli, F.; Casazza, G.; Bacchi Reggiani, M.L.; Cucchetti, A.; Cescon, M.; Festi, D. Role of liver and spleen stiffness in predicting the recurrence of hepatocellular carcinoma after resection. *J. Hepatol.* **2019**, *70*, 440–448. [CrossRef]
85. Hu, X.; Huang, X.; Hou, J.; Ding, L.; Su, C.; Meng, F. Diagnostic accuracy of spleen stiffness to evaluate portal hypertension and esophageal varices in chronic liver disease: A systematic review and meta-analysis. *Eur. Radiol.* **2021**, *31*, 2392–2404. [CrossRef]
86. Kazemi, F.; Kettaneh, A.; N'Kontchou, G.; Pinto, E.; Ganne-Carrie, N.; Trinchet, J.C.; Beaugrand, M. Liver stiffness measurement selects patients with cirrhosis at risk of bearing large oesophageal varices. *J. Hepatol.* **2006**, *45*, 230–235. [CrossRef]
87. Berzigotti, A.; Seijo, S.; Arena, U.; Abraldes, J.G.; Vizzutti, F.; Garcia-Pagan, J.C.; Pinzani, M.; Bosch, J. Elastography, spleen size, and platelet count identify portal hypertension in patients with compensated cirrhosis. *Gastroenterology* **2013**, *144*, 102–111.e1. [CrossRef]
88. De Franchis, R.; Baveno, V.I.F. Expanding consensus in portal hypertension: Report of the Baveno VI Consensus Workshop: Stratifying risk and individualizing care for portal hypertension. *J. Hepatol.* **2015**, *63*, 743–752. [CrossRef] [PubMed]
89. Jiang, H.Y.; Chen, J.; Xia, C.C.; Cao, L.K.; Duan, T.; Song, B. Noninvasive imaging of hepatocellular carcinoma: From diagnosis to prognosis. *World J. Gastroenterol.* **2018**, *24*, 2348–2362. [CrossRef] [PubMed]
90. Marrero, J.A.; Kulik, L.M.; Sirlin, C.B.; Zhu, A.X.; Finn, R.S.; Abecassis, M.M.; Roberts, L.R.; Heimbach, J.K. Diagnosis, Staging, and Management of Hepatocellular Carcinoma: 2018 Practice Guidance by the American Association for the Study of Liver Diseases. *Hepatology* **2018**, *68*, 723–750. [CrossRef] [PubMed]
91. Segura Grau, A.; Valero Lopez, I.; Diaz Rodriguez, N.; Segura Cabral, J.M. Liver ultrasound: Focal lesions and diffuse diseases. *Semergen* **2016**, *42*, 307–314. [CrossRef]
92. Lupsor-Platon, M.; Serban, T.; Silion, A.I.; Tirpe, G.R.; Tirpe, A.; Florea, M. Performance of Ultrasound Techniques and the Potential of Artificial Intelligence in the Evaluation of Hepatocellular Carcinoma and Non-Alcoholic Fatty Liver Disease. *Cancers* **2021**, *13*, 790. [CrossRef]
93. Yoshida, H.; Shiratori, Y.; Moriyama, M.; Arakawa, Y.; Ide, T.; Sata, M.; Inoue, O.; Yano, M.; Tanaka, M.; Fujiyama, S.; et al. Interferon therapy reduces the risk for hepatocellular carcinoma: National surveillance program of cirrhotic and noncirrhotic patients with chronic hepatitis C in Japan. IHIT Study Group. Inhibition of Hepatocarcinogenesis by Interferon Therapy. *Ann. Intern. Med.* **1999**, *131*, 174–181. [CrossRef] [PubMed]
94. Masuzaki, R.; Tateishi, R.; Yoshida, H.; Goto, E.; Sato, T.; Ohki, T.; Imamura, J.; Goto, T.; Kanai, F.; Kato, N.; et al. Prospective risk assessment for hepatocellular carcinoma development in patients with chronic hepatitis C by transient elastography. *Hepatology* **2009**, *49*, 1954–1961. [CrossRef] [PubMed]
95. Kuo, Y.H.; Lu, S.N.; Hung, C.H.; Kee, K.M.; Chen, C.H.; Hu, T.H.; Lee, C.M.; Changchien, C.S.; Wang, J.H. Liver stiffness measurement in the risk assessment of hepatocellular carcinoma for patients with chronic hepatitis. *Hepatol. Int.* **2010**, *4*, 700–706. [CrossRef]
96. Feier, D.; Lupsor Platon, M.; Stefanescu, H.; Badea, R. Transient elastography for the detection of hepatocellular carcinoma in viral C liver cirrhosis. Is there something else than increased liver stiffness? *J. Gastrointestin Liver Dis.* **2013**, *22*, 283–289. [PubMed]
97. Akima, T.; Tamano, M.; Hiraishi, H. Liver stiffness measured by transient elastography is a predictor of hepatocellular carcinoma development in viral hepatitis. *Hepatol. Res.* **2011**, *41*, 965–970. [CrossRef] [PubMed]
98. Wang, H.M.; Hung, C.H.; Lu, S.N.; Chen, C.H.; Lee, C.M.; Hu, T.H.; Wang, J.H. Liver stiffness measurement as an alternative to fibrotic stage in risk assessment of hepatocellular carcinoma incidence for chronic hepatitis C patients. *Liver Int.* **2013**, *33*, 756–761. [CrossRef] [PubMed]
99. Narita, Y.; Genda, T.; Tsuzura, H.; Sato, S.; Kanemitsu, Y.; Ishikawa, S.; Kikuchi, T.; Hirano, K.; Iijima, K.; Wada, R.; et al. Prediction of liver stiffness hepatocellular carcinoma in chronic hepatitis C patients on interferon-based anti-viral therapy. *J. Gastroenterol. Hepatol.* **2014**, *29*, 137–143. [CrossRef]
100. Kim, D.Y.; Song, K.J.; Kim, S.U.; Yoo, E.J.; Park, J.Y.; Ahn, S.H.; Han, K.H. Transient elastography-based risk estimation of hepatitis B virus-related occurrence of hepatocellular carcinoma: Development and validation of a predictive model. *Oncotargets* **2013**, *6*, 1463–1469. [CrossRef]
101. Wong, G.L.; Chan, H.L.; Wong, C.K.; Leung, C.; Chan, C.Y.; Ho, P.P.; Chung, V.C.; Chan, Z.C.; Tse, Y.K.; Chim, A.M.; et al. Liver stiffness-based optimization of hepatocellular carcinoma risk score in patients with chronic hepatitis B. *J. Hepatol.* **2014**, *60*, 339–345. [CrossRef]
102. Lee, H.W.; Ahn, S.H. Prediction models of hepatocellular carcinoma development in chronic hepatitis B patients. *World J. Gastroenterol.* **2016**, *22*, 8314–8321. [CrossRef]
103. Lee, H.W.; Park, S.Y.; Lee, M.; Lee, E.J.; Lee, J.; Kim, S.U.; Park, J.Y.; Kim, D.Y.; Ahn, S.H.; Kim, B.K. An optimized hepatocellular carcinoma prediction model for chronic hepatitis B with well-controlled viremia. *Liver Int.* **2020**, *40*, 1736–1743. [CrossRef] [PubMed]
104. Seo, Y.S.; Jang, B.K.; Um, S.H.; Hwang, J.S.; Han, K.H.; Kim, S.G.; Lee, K.S.; Kim, S.U.; Kim, Y.S.; Lee, J.I. Validation of risk prediction models for the development of HBV-related HCC: A retrospective multi-center 10-year follow-up cohort study. *Oncotarget* **2017**, *8*, 113213–113224. [CrossRef] [PubMed]

105. Cheung, M.C.M.; Walker, A.J.; Hudson, B.E.; Verma, S.; McLauchlan, J.; Mutimer, D.J.; Brown, A.; Gelson, W.T.H.; MacDonald, D.C.; Agarwal, K.; et al. Outcomes after successful direct-acting antiviral therapy for patients with chronic hepatitis C and decompensated cirrhosis. *J. Hepatol.* **2016**, *65*, 741–747. [CrossRef] [PubMed]
106. Romano, A.; Angeli, P.; Piovesan, S.; Noventa, F.; Anastassopoulos, G.; Chemello, L.; Cavalletto, L.; Gambato, M.; Russo, F.P.; Burra, P.; et al. Newly diagnosed hepatocellular carcinoma in patients with advanced hepatitis C treated with DAAs: A prospective population study. *J. Hepatol.* **2018**, *69*, 345–352. [CrossRef]
107. Ioannou, G.N.; Green, P.K.; Berry, K. HCV eradication induced by direct-acting antiviral agents reduces the risk of hepatocellular carcinoma. *J. Hepatol.* **2017**. [CrossRef]
108. Morgan, R.L.; Baack, B.; Smith, B.D.; Yartel, A.; Pitasi, M.; Falck-Ytter, Y. Eradication of hepatitis C virus infection and the development of hepatocellular carcinoma: A meta-analysis of observational studies. *Ann. Intern. Med.* **2013**, *158*, 329–337. [CrossRef]
109. ANRS Collaborative Study Group. Lack of evidence of an effect of direct-acting antivirals on the recurrence of hepatocellular carcinoma: Data from three ANRS cohorts. *J. Hepatol.* **2016**, *65*, 734–740. [CrossRef]
110. Kanwal, F.; Kramer, J.; Asch, S.M.; Chayanupatkul, M.; Cao, Y.; El-Serag, H.B. Risk of Hepatocellular Cancer in HCV Patients Treated With Direct-Acting Antiviral Agents. *Gastroenterology* **2017**, *153*, 996–1005.e1. [CrossRef]
111. Stasi, C.; Sadalla, S.; Carradori, E.; Monti, M.; Petraccia, L.; Madia, F.; Gragnani, L.; Zignego, A.L. Longitudinal evaluation of liver stiffness and outcomes in patients with chronic hepatitis C before and after short- and long-term IFN-free antiviral treatment. *Curr. Med. Res. Opin.* **2020**, *36*, 245–249. [CrossRef]
112. Ravaioli, F.; Conti, F.; Brillanti, S.; Andreone, P.; Mazzella, G.; Buonfiglioli, F.; Serio, I.; Verrucchi, G.; Bacchi Reggiani, M.L.; Colli, A.; et al. Hepatocellular carcinoma risk assessment by the measurement of liver stiffness variations in HCV cirrhotics treated with direct acting antivirals. *Dig. Liver Dis.* **2018**, *50*, 573–579. [CrossRef]
113. Ioannou, G.N.; Green, P.K.; Beste, L.A.; Mun, E.J.; Kerr, K.F.; Berry, K. Development of models estimating the risk of hepatocellular carcinoma after antiviral treatment for hepatitis C. *J. Hepatol.* **2018**, *69*, 1088–1098. [CrossRef] [PubMed]
114. Strazzulla, A.; Iemmolo, R.M.R.; Carbone, E.; Postorino, M.C.; Mazzitelli, M.; De Santis, M.; Di Benedetto, F.; Cristiani, C.M.; Costa, C.; Pisani, V.; et al. The Risk of Hepatocellular Carcinoma After Directly Acting Antivirals for Hepatitis C Virus Treatment in Liver Transplanted Patients: Is It Real? *Hepat. Mon.* **2016**, *16*, e41933. [CrossRef]
115. Masuzaki, R.; Yamashiki, N.; Sugawara, Y.; Yoshida, H.; Tateishi, R.; Tamura, S.; Kaneko, J.; Hasegawa, K.; Kokudo, N.; Makuuchi, M.; et al. Assessment of liver stiffness in patients after living donor liver transplantation by transient elastography. *Scand. J. Gastroenterol.* **2009**, *44*, 1115–1120. [CrossRef]
116. Knop, V.; Hoppe, D.; Welzel, T.; Vermehren, J.; Herrmann, E.; Vermehren, A.; Friedrich-Rust, M.; Sarrazin, C.; Zeuzem, S.; Welker, M.W. Regression of fibrosis and portal hypertension in HCV-associated cirrhosis and sustained virologic response after interferon-free antiviral therapy. *J. Viral. Hepat.* **2016**, *23*, 994–1002. [CrossRef]
117. Ogawa, E.; Furusyo, N.; Toyoda, K.; Takeoka, H.; Maeda, S.; Hayashi, J. The longitudinal quantitative assessment by transient elastography of chronic hepatitis C patients treated with pegylated interferon alpha-2b and ribavirin. *Antivir. Res.* **2009**, *83*, 127–134. [CrossRef] [PubMed]
118. Arima, Y.; Kawabe, N.; Hashimoto, S.; Harata, M.; Nitta, Y.; Murao, M.; Nakano, T.; Shimazaki, H.; Kobayashi, K.; Ichino, N.; et al. Reduction of liver stiffness by interferon treatment in the patients with chronic hepatitis C. *Hepatol. Res.* **2010**, *40*, 383–392. [CrossRef] [PubMed]
119. Macias, J.; del Valle, J.; Rivero, A.; Mira, J.A.; Camacho, A.; Merchante, N.; Perez-Camacho, I.; Neukam, K.; Rivero-Juarez, A.; Mata, R.; et al. Changes in liver stiffness in patients with chronic hepatitis C with and without HIV co-infection treated with pegylated interferon plus ribavirin. *J. Antimicrob. Chemother.* **2010**, *65*, 2204–2211. [CrossRef] [PubMed]
120. Wang, J.H.; Changchien, C.S.; Hung, C.H.; Tung, W.C.; Kee, K.M.; Chen, C.H.; Hu, T.H.; Lee, C.M.; Lu, S.N. Liver stiffness decrease after effective antiviral therapy in patients with chronic hepatitis C: Longitudinal study using FibroScan. *J. Gastroenterol. Hepatol.* **2010**, *25*, 964–969. [CrossRef]
121. Hezode, C.; Castera, L.; Roudot-Thoraval, F.; Bouvier-Alias, M.; Rosa, I.; Roulot, D.; Leroy, V.; Mallat, A.; Pawlotsky, J.M. Liver stiffness diminishes with antiviral response in chronic hepatitis C. *Aliment. Pharm.* **2011**, *34*, 656–663. [CrossRef]
122. Martinez, S.M.; Foucher, J.; Combis, J.M.; Metivier, S.; Brunetto, M.; Capron, D.; Bourliere, M.; Bronowicki, J.P.; Dao, T.; Maynard-Muet, M.; et al. Longitudinal liver stiffness assessment in patients with chronic hepatitis C undergoing antiviral therapy. *PLoS ONE* **2012**, *7*, e47715. [CrossRef]
123. Stasi, C.; Arena, U.; Zignego, A.L.; Corti, G.; Monti, M.; Triboli, E.; Pellegrini, E.; Renzo, S.; Leoncini, L.; Marra, F.; et al. Longitudinal assessment of liver stiffness in patients undergoing antiviral treatment for hepatitis C. *Dig. Liver Dis.* **2013**, *45*, 840–843. [CrossRef]
124. Persico, M.; Rosato, V.; Aglitti, A.; Precone, D.; Corrado, M.; De Luna, A.; Morisco, F.; Camera, S.; Federico, A.; Dallio, M.; et al. Sustained virological response by direct antiviral agents in HCV leads to an early and significant improvement of liver fibrosis. *Antivir. Ther.* **2018**, *23*, 129–138. [CrossRef] [PubMed]
125. Chan, J.; Gogela, N.; Zheng, H.; Lammert, S.; Ajayi, T.; Fricker, Z.; Kim, A.Y.; Robbins, G.K.; Chung, R.T. Direct-Acting Antiviral Therapy for Chronic HCV Infection Results in Liver Stiffness Regression Over 12 Months Post-treatment. *Dig. Dis. Sci.* **2018**, *63*, 486–492. [CrossRef]

126. Giannini, E.G.; Crespi, M.; Demarzo, M.; Bodini, G.; Furnari, M.; Marabotto, E.; Torre, F.; Zentilin, P.; Savarino, V. Improvement in hepatitis C virus patients with advanced, compensated liver disease after sustained virological response to direct acting antivirals. *Eur. J. Clin. Investig.* **2019**, *49*, e13056. [CrossRef] [PubMed]
127. Martinez-Camprecios, J.; Bonis Puig, S.; Pons Delgado, M.; Salcedo Allende, M.T.; Minguez Rosique, B.; Genesca Ferrer, J. Transient elastography in DAA era. Relation between post-SVR LSM and histology. *J. Viral. Hepat.* **2020**, *27*, 453–455. [CrossRef]
128. Knop, V.; Mauss, S.; Goeser, T.; Geier, A.; Zimmermann, T.; Herzer, K.; Postel, N.; Friedrich-Rust, M.; Hofmann, W.P.; German Hepatitis, C.R. Dynamics of liver stiffness by transient elastography in patients with chronic hepatitis C virus infection receiving direct-acting antiviral therapy-Results from the German Hepatitis C-Registry. *J. Viral Hepat.* **2020**, *27*, 690–698. [CrossRef] [PubMed]
129. McPhail, J.; Sims, O.T.; Guo, Y.; Wooten, D.; Herndon, J.S.; Massoud, O.I. Fibrosis improvement in patients with HCV treated with direct-acting antivirals. *Eur. J. Gastroenterol. Hepatol.* **2020**. [CrossRef]
130. Tada, T.; Kumada, T.; Toyoda, H.; Mizuno, K.; Sone, Y.; Kataoka, S.; Hashinokuchi, S. Improvement of liver stiffness in patients with hepatitis C virus infection who received direct-acting antiviral therapy and achieved sustained virological response. *J. Gastroenterol. Hepatol.* **2017**, *32*, 1982–1988. [CrossRef]
131. Bachofner, J.A.; Valli, P.V.; Kroger, A.; Bergamin, I.; Kunzler, P.; Baserga, A.; Braun, D.; Seifert, B.; Moncsek, A.; Fehr, J.; et al. Direct antiviral agent treatment of chronic hepatitis C results in rapid regression of transient elastography and fibrosis markers fibrosis-4 score and aspartate aminotransferase-platelet ratio index. *Liver Int.* **2017**, *37*, 369–376. [CrossRef] [PubMed]
132. Tachi, Y.; Hirai, T.; Kojima, Y.; Ishizu, Y.; Honda, T.; Kuzuya, T.; Hayashi, K.; Ishigami, M.; Goto, H. Liver stiffness reduction correlates with histological characteristics of hepatitis C patients with sustained virological response. *Liver Int.* **2018**, *38*, 59–67. [CrossRef]
133. Rockey, D.C. Fibrosis reversal after hepatitis C virus elimination. *Curr. Opin. Gastroenterol.* **2019**, *35*, 137–144. [CrossRef] [PubMed]
134. D'Ambrosio, R.; Aghemo, A.; Rumi, M.G.; Ronchi, G.; Donato, M.F.; Paradis, V.; Colombo, M.; Bedossa, P. A morphometric and immunohistochemical study to assess the benefit of a sustained virological response in hepatitis C virus patients with cirrhosis. *Hepatology* **2012**, *56*, 532–543. [CrossRef] [PubMed]
135. Goossens, N.; Negro, F. Is genotype 3 of the hepatitis C virus the new villain? *Hepatology* **2014**, *59*, 2403–2412. [CrossRef] [PubMed]
136. Asselah, T.; Rubbia-Brandt, L.; Marcellin, P.; Negro, F. Steatosis in chronic hepatitis C: Why does it really matter? *Gut* **2006**, *55*, 123–130. [CrossRef]
137. Castera, L.; Hezode, C.; Roudot-Thoraval, F.; Bastie, A.; Zafrani, E.S.; Pawlotsky, J.M.; Dhumeaux, D. Worsening of steatosis is an independent factor of fibrosis progression in untreated patients with chronic hepatitis C and paired liver biopsies. *Gut* **2003**, *52*, 288–292. [CrossRef] [PubMed]
138. Kurosaki, M.; Hosokawa, T.; Matsunaga, K.; Hirayama, I.; Tanaka, T.; Sato, M.; Yasui, Y.; Tamaki, N.; Ueda, K.; Tsuchiya, K.; et al. Hepatic steatosis in chronic hepatitis C is a significant risk factor for developing hepatocellular carcinoma independent of age, sex, obesity, fibrosis stage and response to interferon therapy. *Hepatol. Res.* **2010**, *40*, 870–877. [CrossRef]
139. Leandro, G.; Mangia, A.; Hui, J.; Fabris, P.; Rubbia-Brandt, L.; Colloredo, G.; Adinolfi, L.E.; Asselah, T.; Jonsson, J.R.; Smedile, A.; et al. Relationship between steatosis, inflammation, and fibrosis in chronic hepatitis C: A meta-analysis of individual patient data. *Gastroenterology* **2006**, *130*, 1636–1642. [CrossRef]
140. Fartoux, L.; Chazouilleres, O.; Wendum, D.; Poupon, R.; Serfaty, L. Impact of steatosis on progression of fibrosis in patients with mild hepatitis C. *Hepatology* **2005**, *41*, 82–87. [CrossRef]
141. Stern, C.; Castera, L. Non-invasive diagnosis of hepatic steatosis. *Hepatol. Int.* **2017**, *11*, 70–78. [CrossRef]
142. Hernaez, R.; Lazo, M.; Bonekamp, S.; Kamel, I.; Brancati, F.L.; Guallar, E.; Clark, J.M. Diagnostic accuracy and reliability of ultrasonography for the detection of fatty liver: A meta-analysis. *Hepatology* **2011**, *54*, 1082–1090. [CrossRef]
143. Webb, M.; Yeshua, H.; Zelber-Sagi, S.; Santo, E.; Brazowski, E.; Halpern, Z.; Oren, R. Diagnostic value of a computerized hepatorenal index for sonographic quantification of liver steatosis. *AJR Am. J. Roentgenol.* **2009**, *192*, 909–914. [CrossRef]
144. Jeon, S.K.; Joo, I.; Kim, S.Y.; Jang, J.K.; Park, J.; Park, H.S.; Lee, E.S.; Lee, J.M. Quantitative ultrasound radiofrequency data analysis for the assessment of hepatic steatosis using the controlled attenuation parameter as a reference standard. *Ultrasonography* **2021**, *40*, 136–146. [CrossRef]
145. Sasso, M.; Tengher-Barna, I.; Ziol, M.; Miette, V.; Fournier, C.; Sandrin, L.; Poupon, R.; Cardoso, A.C.; Marcellin, P.; Douvin, C.; et al. Novel controlled attenuation parameter for noninvasive assessment of steatosis using Fibroscan((R)): Validation in chronic hepatitis C. *J. Viral. Hepat.* **2012**, *19*, 244–253. [CrossRef]
146. Ferraioli, G.; Tinelli, C.; Lissandrin, R.; Zicchetti, M.; Dal Bello, B.; Filice, G.; Filice, C. Controlled attenuation parameter for evaluating liver steatosis in chronic viral hepatitis. *World J. Gastroenterol.* **2014**, *20*, 6626–6631. [CrossRef]
147. De Ledinghen, V.; Vergniol, J.; Foucher, J.; Merrouche, W.; le Bail, B. Non-invasive diagnosis of liver steatosis using controlled attenuation parameter (CAP) and transient elastography. *Liver Int.* **2012**, *32*, 911–918. [CrossRef]
148. Mi, Y.Q.; Shi, Q.Y.; Xu, L.; Shi, R.F.; Liu, Y.G.; Li, P.; Shen, F.; Lu, W.; Fan, J.G. Controlled attenuation parameter for noninvasive assessment of hepatic steatosis using Fibroscan(R): Validation in chronic hepatitis B. *Dig. Dis. Sci.* **2015**, *60*, 243–251. [CrossRef]
149. Wang, Y.; Fan, Q.; Wang, T.; Wen, J.; Wang, H.; Zhang, T. Controlled attenuation parameter for assessment of hepatic steatosis grades: A diagnostic meta-analysis. *Int. J. Clin. Exp. Med.* **2015**, *8*, 17654–17663. [PubMed]

150. Pu, K.; Wang, Y.; Bai, S.; Wei, H.; Zhou, Y.; Fan, J.; Qiao, L. Diagnostic accuracy of controlled attenuation parameter (CAP) as a non-invasive test for steatosis in suspected non-alcoholic fatty liver disease: A systematic review and meta-analysis. *BMC Gastroenterol.* **2019**, *19*, 51. [CrossRef]
151. Moret, A.; Boursier, J.; Houssel Debry, P.; Riou, J.; Crouan, A.; Dubois, M.; Michalak Provost, S.; Aube, C.; Paisant, A. Evaluation of the Hepatorenal B-Mode Ratio and the "Controlled Attenuation Parameter" for the Detection and Grading of Steatosis. *Ultraschall Med.* **2020**. [CrossRef]
152. Rout, G.; Nayak, B.; Patel, A.H.; Gunjan, D.; Singh, V.; Kedia, S. Therapy with Oral Directly Acting Agents in Hepatitis C Infection Is Associated with Reduction in Fibrosis and Increase in Hepatic Steatosis on Transient Elastography. *J. Clin. Exp. Hepatol.* **2019**, *9*, 207–214. [CrossRef] [PubMed]
153. Ogasawara, N.; Kobayashi, M.; Akuta, N.; Kominami, Y.; Fujiyama, S.; Kawamura, Y.; Sezaki, H.; Hosaka, T.; Suzuki, F.; Saitoh, S.; et al. Serial changes in liver stiffness and controlled attenuation parameter following direct-acting antiviral therapy against hepatitis C virus genotype 1b. *J. Med. Virol.* **2018**, *90*, 313–319. [CrossRef] [PubMed]
154. Kobayashi, N.; Iijima, H.; Tada, T.; Kumada, T.; Yoshida, M.; Aoki, T.; Nishimura, T.; Nakano, C.; Takata, R.; Yoh, K.; et al. Changes in liver stiffness and steatosis among patients with hepatitis C virus infection who received direct-acting antiviral therapy and achieved sustained virological response. *Eur. J. Gastroenterol. Hepatol.* **2018**, *30*, 546–551. [CrossRef] [PubMed]
155. Shimizu, K.; Soroida, Y.; Sato, M.; Hikita, H.; Kobayashi, T.; Endo, M.; Sato, M.; Gotoh, H.; Iwai, T.; Tateishi, R.; et al. Eradication of hepatitis C virus is associated with the attenuation of steatosis as evaluated using a controlled attenuation parameter. *Sci. Rep.* **2018**, *8*, 7845. [CrossRef] [PubMed]
156. Sung, J.C.; Wyatt, B.E.; Perumalswami, P.V.; Branch, A.D. Response to 'hepatitis C cure improved patient-reported outcomes in patients with and without liver fibrosis in a prospective study at a large urban medical center'. *J. Viral. Hepat.* **2020**, *27*, 1502–1503. [CrossRef] [PubMed]
157. Ferraioli, G.; Filice, C.; Castera, L.; Choi, B.I.; Sporea, I.; Wilson, S.R.; Cosgrove, D.; Dietrich, C.F.; Amy, D.; Bamber, J.C.; et al. WFUMB guidelines and recommendations for clinical use of ultrasound elastography: Part 3: Liver. *Ultrasound Med. Biol.* **2015**, *41*, 1161–1179. [CrossRef] [PubMed]

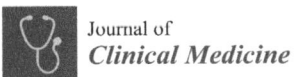 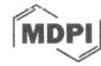

Article

Effectiveness and Safety of Pangenotypic Regimens in the Most Difficult to Treat Population of Genotype 3 HCV Infected Cirrhotics

Dorota Zarębska-Michaluk [1,*], Jerzy Jaroszewicz [2], Anna Parfieniuk-Kowerda [3], Ewa Janczewska [4], Dorota Dybowska [5], Małgorzata Pawłowska [5], Waldemar Halota [5], Włodzimierz Mazur [6], Beata Lorenc [7], Justyna Janocha-Litwin [8], Krzysztof Simon [8], Anna Piekarska [9], Hanna Berak [10], Jakub Klapaczyński [11], Piotr Stępień [1], Barbara Sobala-Szczygieł [2], Jolanta Citko [12], Łukasz Socha [13], Magdalena Tudrujek-Zdunek [14], Krzysztof Tomasiewicz [14], Marek Sitko [15], Beata Dobracka [16], Rafał Krygier [17], Jolanta Białkowska-Warzecha [18], Łukasz Laurans [13,19] and Robert Flisiak [3]

Citation: Zarębska-Michaluk, D.; Jaroszewicz, J.; Parfieniuk-Kowerda, A.; Janczewska, E.; Dybowska, D.; Pawłowska, M.; Halota, W.; Mazur, W.; Lorenc, B.; Janocha-Litwin, J.; et al. Effectiveness and Safety of Pangenotypic Regimens in the Most Difficult to Treat Population of Genotype 3 HCV Infected Cirrhotics. *J. Clin. Med.* 2021, 10, 3280. https://doi.org/10.3390/jcm10153280

Academic Editors: Maria Carla Liberto and Giovanni Tarantino

Received: 13 June 2021
Accepted: 22 July 2021
Published: 25 July 2021

Publisher's Note: MDPI stays neutral with regard to jurisdictional claims in published maps and institutional affiliations.

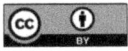

Copyright: © 2021 by the authors. Licensee MDPI, Basel, Switzerland. This article is an open access article distributed under the terms and conditions of the Creative Commons Attribution (CC BY) license (https://creativecommons.org/licenses/by/4.0/).

1 Department of Infectious Diseases, Jan Kochanowski University, 25-317 Kielce, Poland; p_stepien@interia.pl
2 Department of Infectious Diseases and Hepatology, Medical University of Silesia, 40-055 Katowice, Poland; jerzy.jr@gmail.com (J.J.); sobala.szczygiel@op.pl (B.S.-S.)
3 Department of Infectious Diseases and Hepatology, Medical University of Białystok, 15-540 Białystok, Poland; anna.parfieniuk@gmail.com (A.P.-K.); robert.flisiak1@gmail.com (R.F.)
4 Department of Basic Medical Sciences, Faculty of Health Sciences in Bytom, Medical University of Silesia, 41-902 Bytom, Poland; e.janczewska@poczta.fm
5 Department of Infectious Diseases and Hepatology, Collegium Medicum, Nicolaus Copernicus University, 87-030 Bydgoszcz, Poland; d.dybowska@wsoz.pl (D.D.); mpawlowska@cm.umk.pl (M.P.); w.halota@wsoz.pl (W.H.)
6 Clinical Department of Infectious Diseases, Medical University of Silesia in Katowice, 41-500 Chorzów, Poland; wlodek.maz@gmail.com
7 Pomeranian Center of Infectious Diseases, Medical University Gdańsk, 80-214 Gdańsk, Poland; lormar@gumed.edu.pl
8 Department of Infectious Diseases, Medical University Wrocław, 50-367 Wrocław, Poland; justynajanocha@o2.pl (J.J.-L.); krzysimon@gmail.com (K.S.)
9 Department of Infectious Diseases, Medical University of Łódź, 90-419 Łódź, Poland; annapiekar@gmail.com
10 Hospital for Infectious Diseases in Warszawa, 02-091 Warsaw, Poland; hberak@wp.pl
11 Department of Internal Medicine and Hepatology, Central Clinical Hospital of the Ministry of Internal Affairs and Administration, 00-241 Warszawa, Poland; klapaj@gmail.com
12 Medical Practice of Infections, Regional Hospital, 10-561 Olsztyn, Poland; citkoj@wss.olsztyn.pl
13 Department of Infectious Diseases, Hepatology and Liver Transplantation, Pomeranian Medical University, 71-455 Szczecin, Poland; theville@wp.pl (Ł.S.); asklepiada@wp.pl (Ł.L.)
14 Department of Infectious Diseases, Medical University of Lublin, 20-059 Lublin, Poland; magdalena.tudrujek@gmail.com (M.T.-Z.); tomaskdr@poczta.fm (K.T.)
15 Department of Infectious and Tropical Diseases, Jagiellonian University, 31-088 Kraków, Poland; sitkomar@o2.pl
16 MED-FIX, 53-522 Wrocław, Poland; dobrackab@gmail.com
17 Outpatients Hepatology Department, State University of Applied Sciences, 62-510 Konin, Poland; rafalkrygier@gmail.com
18 Department of Infectious and Liver Diseases, Medical University Łódź, 90-419 Łódź, Poland; jbialkowska@pro.onet.pl
19 Multidisciplinary Regional Hospital, 66-418 Gorzów Wielkopolski, Poland
* Correspondence: dorota1010@tlen.pl; Tel.: +48-66-244-1465; Fax: +48-41-368-2262

Abstract: There is still limited data available from real-world experience studies on the pangenotypic regimens in patients with genotype (GT) 3 hepatitis C virus (HCV) infection and liver cirrhosis. The current study aimed to evaluate the efficacy and safety of pangenotypic regimens in this difficult-to-treat population. A total of 236 patients with mean age 52.3 ± 11.3 years and male predominance (72%) selected from EpiTer-2 database were included in the analysis; 72% of them were treatment-naïve. The majority of patients (55%) received the combination of sofosbuvir/velpatasvir (SOF/VEL), 71 without and 58 with ribavirin (RBV), whereas the remaining 107 individuals were assigned to glecaprevir/pibrentasvir (GLE/PIB). The effectiveness of the treatment following GLE/PIB and

SOF/VEL regimens (96% and 93%) was higher compared to SOF/VEL + RBV option (79%). The univariate analysis demonstrated the significantly lower sustained virologic response in males, in patients with baseline HCV RNA ≥ 1,000,000 IU/mL, and among those who failed previous DAA-based therapy. The multivariate logistic regression analysis recognized only the male gender and presence of ascites at baseline as the independent factors of non-response to treatment. It should be emphasized that despite the availability of pangenotypic, strong therapeutic options, GT3 infected patients with cirrhosis still remain difficult-to-treat, especially those with hepatic impairment and DAA-experienced.

Keywords: hepatitis C; genotype 3; liver cirrhosis; pangenotypic

1. Introduction

Chronic infection with the hepatitis C virus (HCV) seems to be one of the significant health problems worldwide. Approximately 71 million people are affected globally, of whom 400,000 died annually due to the consequences of the disease [1]. The most severe complications of chronic hepatitis C (CHC) with a risk of death are liver cirrhosis and hepatocellular carcinoma (HCC). The development of liver fibrosis leading to cirrhosis occurs in nearly 20% of patients, and, on average, two decades of HCV infection are needed for this [2]. However, the rate of progression of fibrosis varies between different patients and depends on both viral and host predictors [2]. Male gender, the age of infection over 40 years, coinfection with hepatitis B virus (HBV) and human immunodeficiency virus (HIV), obesity, alcohol abuse are listed among variables related to the infected person, whereas the most important viral predictor for the accelerated fibrosis is genotype (GT) 3 HCV, which is second in frequency worldwide accounting for 25–30% all HCV cases [3–6]. In the era of interferon (IFN) based therapy, patients with liver cirrhosis had limited access to antiviral treatment due to safety issues and low effectiveness [7]. The implementation of the IFN-free DAA regimens has removed those safety-related limitations, but sofosbuvir (SOF) plus ribavirin (RBV), the only option available initially for GT3 patients, had still relatively low efficacy as compared to the cure rate achieved with DAA therapies in other GTs-infected individuals and treatment with daclatasvir (DCV) plus SOF was not available worldwide [8–10]. Therefore, at the beginning of the IFN-free era, cirrhotics infected with GT3 were assumed to be the most difficult-to-treat patients with CHC. The latest development in the antiviral treatment of this subpopulation was the registration of pangenotypic regimens. According to the recent guidelines, two options are recommended in patients with liver cirrhosis in the course of GT3 infection, the combination of protease inhibitor glecaprevir (GLE) with the inhibitor of non-structural protein 5A (NS5A) pibrentasvir (PIB), and SOF, polymerase inhibitor with velpatasvir (VEL), acting by inhibition of NS5A HCV [11–14]. However, available data in this population are based on limited studies, which usually included a small number of patients. The current study aimed to evaluate the efficacy of pangenotypic regimens in patients with liver cirrhosis infected with GT3 in the real-world experience.

2. Materials and Methods

The analyzed population consisted of CHC patients with liver cirrhosis infected with GT3 HCV selected from EpiTer-2 database. This sizeable national project supported by the Polish Association of Epidemiologists and Infectiologists includes 13,554 individuals treated with DAA regimens in 22 Polish hepatology centers between 1 July 2015 and 31 December 2020. Clinical data, including the severity of liver disease, the presence of the extrahepatic manifestations, coexisting medical conditions, concomitant medications, coinfections, the history of previous antiviral treatment and currently used regimen, and laboratory parameters were collected at baseline.

The severity of liver disease was assessed based on the non-invasive fibrosis evaluation either by transient elastography (TE) or shear-wave elastography (SWE), and cirrhosis was diagnosed according to recommendations of the European Association for the Study of the Liver (EASL) if liver stiffness ≥13 kilopascals corresponding to a METAVIR score of F4 [11]. In addition, cirrhotic patients were assessed for the oesophageal varices, past or present hepatic decompensation, history of liver transplantation, and scored in Child-Pugh (CP) scale and Model of End Stage Liver Disease (MELD).

HCV RNA was measured at baseline, at the end of treatment (EOT), and 12 weeks after therapy completion. The efficacy endpoint was sustained virologic response (SVR) defined as undetectable HCV RNA post-treatment week 12. The intent-to-treat (ITT) population included all patients who initiated the treatment, whereas per-protocol (PP) analysis was performed after excluding lost follow-up patients considered to be a non-virologic failure. Safety data in terms of adverse events (AE) and deaths were collected during the treatment course and in the 12-weeks follow-up period. Data were collected retrospectively and submitted by an online questionnaire administered by Tiba sp. z o.o.

Statistical Analysis

Results were expressed as mean (SD) or number (percentage). A p value less than 0.05 was considered significant. The significance of differences was calculated by the χ^2 or Fisher exact tests for nominal variables and by the Mann–Whitney test and the Kruskal-Wallis analysis of variance for continuous variables. Univariable comparisons were calculated using the GraphPad Prism 5.1 software (GraphPad Software, Inc., La Jolla, CA, USA). The general logistic regression model was performed with SVR as the dependent variable. Among independent variables tested for the best model were age, sex, response to previous therapy, anamnesis of hepatic decompensation, baseline ascites, serum bilirubin, albumin, platelets, and HCV RNA. Logistic regression models were calculated by use of Statistica 13.0 (TIBCO Software Inc., Palo Alto, CA, USA).

3. Results

A total of 236 patients with liver cirrhosis infected with GT3 with mean age 52.3 ± 11.3 years and male predominance (72%) treated with pangenotypic regimens were included in the analysis. One hundred and seven (45%) were assigned to GLE/PIB, whereas the remaining 129 patients received SOF/VEL including 58 on the regimen with RBV. The choice of the therapeutic option was made by treating physicians in line with guidelines of the Polish Group of Experts for HCV and the recommendations of the National Health Fund, taking into consideration patients' characteristics and drug labels.

No significant differences in demographic variables, as well as rates of comorbidities and concomitant medications, were observed between patients treated with two pangenotypic regimens (Table 1).

Table 1. Baseline characteristics of GT3 HCV infected patients with liver cirrhosis treated with pangenotypic regimens.

Parameter	GLE/PIB $n = 107$	SOF/VEL $n = 71$	SOV/VEL + RBV $n = 58$	p
Gender, females/males, n (%)	30 (28)/77 (72)	23 (32.4)/48 (67.6)	13 (22.4)/45 (77.6)	0.45
Age [years] mean (SD)	51.8 (10.6)	53.2 (12.5)	53.0 (11.3)	0.96
BMI mean (SD)	27.8 (4.7)	27.5 (4.8)	29.0 (5.6)	0.31
Comorbidities, n (%)	75 (70.1)	50 (70.4)	40 (69)	0.98
Concomitant medications, n (%)	70 (65.4)	47 (66.2)	45 (77.6)	0.24
ALT IU/L, mean (SD)	141 (116)	132 (92)	106 (70)	0.17
Bilirubin mg/dL, mean (SD)	1.0 (0.6)	0.8 (0.4)	1.3 (0.8)	0.003
Albumin g/dL, mean (SD)	3.9 (0.5)	3.9 (0.5)	3.7 (0.5)	0.02
Creatinine mg/dL, mean (SD)	0.9 (0.6)	0.8 (0.2)	0.8 (0.2)	0.74
Hemoglobin g/dL, mean (SD)	14.4 (1.8)	14.5 (1.5)	13.9 (1.7)	0.27
Platelets, ×1000/μL, mean (SD)	139 (82)	128 (54)	95 (53)	<0.001
HCV RNA × 10^6 IU/mL, mean (SD)	2.17 (4.31)	1.45 (1.79)	1.49 (2.29)	0.62

HCV, hepatitis C virus; GLE, glecaprevir; PIB, pibrentasvir; SOF, sofosbuvir; VEL, velpatasvir; RBV, ribavirin; SD, standard deviation; BMI, body mass index; ALT, alanine transaminase; HCV RNA, ribonucleic acid of hepatitis C virus.

Significantly higher bilirubin concentration, lower albumin level, and platelet count were found among patients treated with SOF/VEL + RBV. In addition, in this subpopulation, a significantly higher percentage of those with past and present hepatic decompensation were observed, and a higher rate of individuals in category B of the Child-Pugh scale (Table 2).

Table 2. Characteristics of the liver disease in GT3 HCV infected patients with liver cirrhosis treated with pangenotypic regimens.

Parameter	GLE/PIB $n = 107$	SOF/VEL $n = 71$	SOF/VEL + RBV $n = 58$	p
History of hepatic decompensation, n (%)				
Number of patients	2 (1.8)	3 (4.2)	9 (15.5)	0.001
Ascites	1 (0.9)	3 (4.2)	9 (15.5)	<0.001
Encephalopathy	1 (0.9)	1 (1.4)	1 (1.7)	0.91
Documented esophageal varices, n (%)	22 (20.6)	11 (15.5)	12 (20.7)	0.66
Hepatic decompensation at baseline, n (%)				
Moderate ascites—responded to diuretics	0	1 (1.4)	6 (10.3)	<0.001
Tense ascites—not responded to diuretics	0	0	0	na
Encephalopathy	0	0	0	na
HCC history, n (%)	4 (3.7)	2 (2.8)	1 (1.7)	0.76
OLTx history, n (%)	0	0	0	na
Child-Pugh, n (%)				
A	102 (95.3)	70 (98.6)	53 (91.4)	0.15
B	5 (4.7)	1 (1.4)	5 (8.6)	0.15
C	0	0	0	na
MELD, n (%)				
<15	100 (93.6)	67 (94.4)	58 (100)	0.15
15–18	3 (2.8)	1 (1.4)	0	na
19–20	2 (1.8)	1 (1.4)	0	na
>20	1 (0.9)	0	0	na
No data	1 (0.9)	2 (2.8)	0	na
HBV coinfection (HBsAg+), n (%)	2 (1.8)	3 (4.2)	0	0.24
HIV coinfection, n (%)	7 (6.5)	9 12.7)	3 (5.1)	0.22

HCV, hepatitis C virus; GLE, glecaprevir; PIB, pibrentasvir; SOF, sofosbuvir; VEL, velpatasvir; RBV, ribavirin; hepatocellular carcinoma; OLTx, orthotopic liver transplantation; MELD, Model End-Stage Liver Disease; HBV, hepatitis B virus; HBsAg+, hepatitis B surface antigen; HIV, human immunodeficiency virus.

The significantly lower percentage of patients treated with SOF/VEL+RBV were treatment-naïve as compared to SOF/VEL and GLE/PIB regimens, 55.2%, 77.5%, and 77.6%, respectively. The relapse rate was the highest among those assigned to SOF/VEL + RBV option, and SOF + RBV was the most frequently used previous regimen in all subpopulations. A total of 30 patients were nonresponders to previous DAA-containing therapy without IFN, and eight of them were treated in the past with NS5A inhibitors. Six of those who previously failed NS5A-containing regimens were treated with SOF/VEL + RBV; the remaining two patients received GLE/PIB in re-therapy.

The majority of patients on the GLE/PIB option received a 12-weeks regimen (60.7%); more than half (55%) of those assigned to SOF/VEL therapy were treated for 12 weeks without RBV (Table 3).

A total of 211 patients achieved an SVR corresponding to 89.4% in the ITT analysis, and after exclusion of four patients lost to follow-up, 91% in the PP analysis. The SVR rate was significantly higher among patients treated with GLE/PIB compared to those receiving SOF/VEL ± RBV both in ITT and PP analyses, 94.4% vs. 85.3% (p = 0.03), and 96.2% vs. 86.6%, (p = 0.01), respectively (Figure 1).

Table 3. Previous and current treatment characteristics of GT3 HCV infected patients with liver cirrhosis treated with pangenotypic regimens.

Parameter	GLE/PIB n = 107	SOF/VEL n = 71	SOF/VEL + RBV n = 58	p
History of previous therapy, n (%)				
Treatment-naïve	83 (77.6)	55 (77.5)	32 (55.2)	0.004
Nonresponder	3 (2.8)	3 (4.2)	4 (6.9)	0.46
Relapser	16 (14.9)	12 (16.9)	20 (34.5)	0.008
Discontinuation due to safety reasons	0	0	1 (1.7)	na
Unknown type of response	5 (4.7)	1 (1.4)	1 (1.7)	0.37
Previous regimen in patients with treatment failure, n (%)	n = 24	n = 16	n = 26	
PegIFNα + RBV	5 (20.8)	6 (37.5)	4 (15.4)	0.24
SOF + PegIFNα + RBV	4 (16.7)	3 (19)	4 (15.4)	0.96
SOF + RBV	12 (50)	7 (43.8)	11 (42.3)	0.85
SOF/VEL ± RBV	2 (8.3)	0	0	na
SOF/LDV	0	0	1 (3.8)	na
GLE/PIB	0	0	4 (15.4)	na
Other	0	0	2 (7.7) *	na
No data	1 (4.2)	0	0	na
Current treatment regimens, n (%)				
GLE/PIB, 8 weeks	20 (18.7)	na	na	
GLE/PIB, 12 weeks	65 (60.7)	na	na	
GLE/PIB, 16 weeks	22 (20.6)	na	na	
SOF/VEL, 12 weeks	na	71 (100)	na	
SOF/VEL + RBV, 12 weeks	na	na	48 (82.7)	na
SOF/VEL + RBV, 24 weeks	na	na	10 (16.3)	

HCV, hepatitis C virus; GLE, glecaprevir; PIB, pibrentasvir; SOF, sofosbuvir; VEL, velpatasvir; RBV, ribavirin; PegIFNα, pegylated interferon alpha; LDV, ledipasvir. * IFNα + RBV, Uprifosbuvir + Grazoprevir + Elbasvir/Ruzasvir.

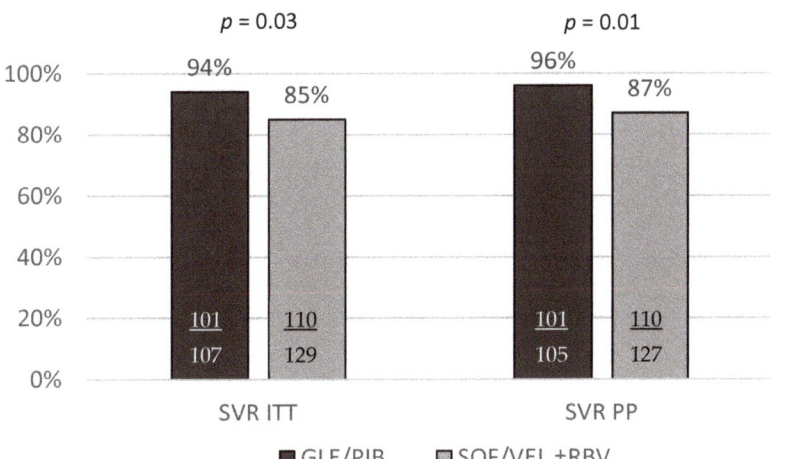

Figure 1. The comparison of the SVR rates between GT3 HCV infected patients with liver cirrhosis treated with GLE/PIB and SOF/VEL ± RBV regimens.

The detailed comparison of an SVR rates revealed no significant difference between GLE/PIB and SOF/VEL regimens, whereas cirrhotics on SOV/VEL + RBV option had significantly lower SVR as compared to both remaining options, 77.6% vs. 91.5% ($p = 0.04$), vs. 94.4% ($p = 0.002$), and 78.9% vs. 92.9% ($p = 0.003$), vs. 96.2% ($p = 0.001$), in ITT and PP analysis, respectively (Figure 2).

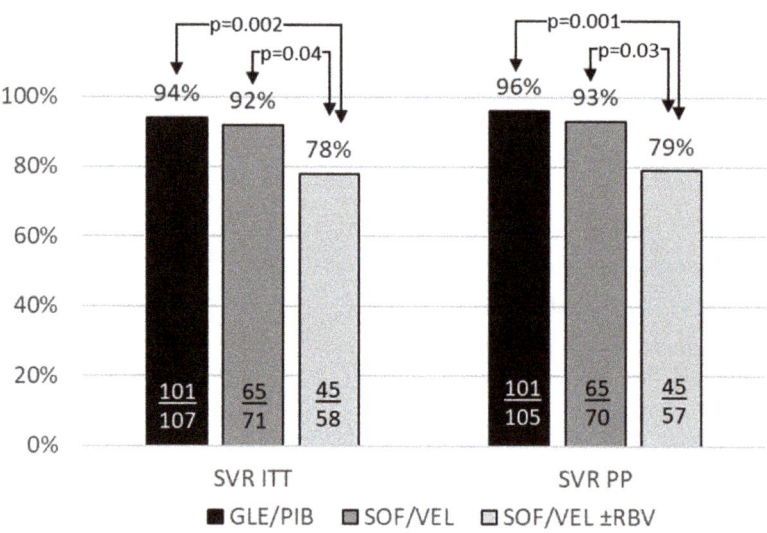

Figure 2. The effectiveness of the GLE/PIB, SOF/VEL, and SOF/VEL + RBV options in GT3 infected patients with liver cirrhosis.

A total of twenty-three virologic failures were documented, 6 on GLE/PIB and 17 on SOF/VEL ± RBV regimen (Tables 4 and 5).

Table 4. Characteristics of 6 virologic failures to GLE/PIB regimen.

Patient	Age	CP	Regimen	History of Previous Therapy	Baseline HCV RNA IU/mL	Treatment Course	EOT	Comment (Possible Reason for Non-Response)
Female 1	56	A	GLE/PIB 12	treatment-naive	2,518,022	according to plan	TD	
Male 1	48	A	GLE/PIB 8	treatment-naive	942,000	according to plan	TND	
Male 2	51	A	GLE/PIB 8	treatment-naive	1,621,033	according to plan	TD	
Male 3	52	A	GLE/PIB 8	treatment-naive	1,483,266	according to plan	TND	
Male 4	30	A	GLE/PIB 12	treatment-naive	1,580,000	according to plan	TND	
Male 5	54	A	GLE/PIB 16	relapse (SOF + RBV)	4,030,000	according to plan	TND	DAA failure

GLE, glecaprevir; PIB, pibrentasvir; CP, Child-Pugh scale; HCV RNA, ribonucleic acid of hepatitis C virus; EOT, end of treatment; TD, target detected; TND, target not detected; SOF, sofosbuvir; RBV, ribavirin; DAA, direct-acting antivirals.

All of them were scored as category A on the CP scale; one experienced RBV dose reduction, and another one discontinued therapy by his own decision. Twenty-one of them were males, and nine were nonresponders to previous DAA-containing therapy, of whom two were treated in the past with pegylated IFN alpha (pegIFNα) + RBV + SOF, 4 received SOF + RBV, two another with GLE/PIB and one patient as a participant of the clinical trial did not respond to uprifosbuvir + grazoprevir + elbasvir/ruzasvir.

A significantly higher rate of males (91.3% vs. 69.4%, $p = 0.03$) was documented in GT3-infected nonresponders to pangenotypic regimens than those who achieved an SVR (Table 6).

The univariate analysis demonstrated the significantly lower SVR in males, in patients with baseline HCV RNA $\geq$ 1,000,000 IU/mL compared to <1,000,000 IU/mL, and among those who failed previous DAA-based therapy (Table 7).

The multivariate logistic regression analysis recognized the male gender and presence of ascites at baseline as the independent factors of non-response to pangenotypic treatment (Table 8).

Table 5. Characteristics of 17 virologic failures to SOF/VEL ± RBV regimen.

Patient	Age	CP	Regimen	History of Previous Therapy	Baseline HCV RNA IU/mL	Treatment Course	EOT	Comment (Possible Reason for Non-Response)
Female 1	44	A	SOF/VEL + RBV 12	treatment-naive	3,560,000	RBV dose reduction	TD	
Male 1	50	A	SOF/VEL 12	relapse (SOF + RBV)	2,190,000	according to plan	TND	DAA failure
Male 2	54	A	SOF/VEL 12	relapse (SOF + RBV)	5279	according to plan	TND	DAA failure
Male 3	49	A	SOF/VEL 12	treatment-naive	1,014,206	according to plan	TD	
Male 4	38	A	SOF/VEL 12	treatment-naive	4,910,000	according to plan	TD	
Male 5	50	A	SOF/VEL 12	treatment-naive	70,000	according to plan	TD	
Male 6	58	A	SOF/VEL + RBV 12	treatment-naive	1,620,000	according to plan	TND	
Male 7	54	A	SOF/VEL + RBV 12	relapse (SOF + RBV)	667,000	according to plan	TND	DAA failure
Male 8	53	A	SOF/VEL + RBV 12	relapse (PR + SOF)	261,902	according to plan	TND	DAA failure
Male 9	29	A	SOF/VEL + RBV 12	relapse (PR + SOF)	534,255	according to plan	TND	DAA failure
Male 10	50	A	SOF/VEL + RBV 12	relapse (Uprifosbuvir + Grazoprevir + Elbasvir or Ruzasvir)	2,230,000	according to plan	TND	DAA failure
Male 11	58	A	SOF/VEL + RBV 12	relapse (GLE/PIB)	1,270,000	according to plan	TND	DAA failure
Male 12	51	A	SOF/VEL + RBV 12	treatment-naive	1,790,000	according to plan	TND	
Male 13	70	A	SOF/VEL + RBV 12	treatment-naive	2,420,000	according to plan	TND	
Male 14	52	A	SOF/VEL + RBV 12	treatment-naive	1,220,000	according to plan	TD	
Male 15	73	A	SOF/VEL + RBV 12	treatment-naive	4,270,000	discontinued	TD	Treatment discontinuation
Male 16	56	A	SOF/VEL + RBV 24	relapse (GLE/PIB)	1,080,000	according to plan	TND	DAA failure

SOF, sofosbuvir; VEL, velpatasvir; RBV, ribavirin; CP, Child-Pugh scale; HCV RNA, ribonucleic acid of hepatitis C virus; EOT, end of treatment; TD, target detected; TND, target not detected; DAA, direct-acting antivirals; PR, PegIFNα + RBV; GLE, glecaprevir; PIB, pibrentasvir.

Table 6. Virologic nonresponders vs. responders to pangenotypic regimens.

Parameter	Virologic Nonresponders n = 23	Responders n = 209	p
Gender, females/males, n (%)	2 (8.7)/21 (91.3)	64 (30.6)/145 (69.4)	0.03
Age [years] mean (SD)	51.3 (10)	52.8 (11.5)	0.67
BMI mean (SD)	28.8 (4.6)	28.0 (5.1)	0.44
Any comorbidity, n (%)	16 (69.6)	147 (70.3)	1.00
Concomitant medications, n (%)	18 (78.3)	143 (68.4)	0.47
HBV coinfection (HBsAg+), n (%)	0	5 (2.4)	1.00
HIV coinfection, n (%)	2 (8.7)	16 (7.7)	0.69
Liver stiffness kPa, mean (SD)	28 (13.3)	28.8 (17.5)	0.71
History of hepatic decompensation, n (%)	3 (13)	11 (5.3)	0.15
HCC history, n (%)	1 (4.3)	6 (2.9)	0.52
Hepatic decompensation at baseline, n (%)	2 (8.7)	5 (2.4)	0.14
Child-Pugh B, n (%)	0	10 (4.8)	0.60
Treatment-experienced, n (%)	9 (39.1)	54 (25.8)	0.22
IFN-free DAA-experienced, n (%)	7 (30.4)	29 (13.9)	0.06
ALT IU/L, mean (SD)	143 (85)	129 (102)	0.24
Bilirubin mg/dL, mean (SD)	1.15 (0.38)	1.0 (0.64)	0.01
Albumin g/dL, mean (SD)	3.87 (0.55)	3.86 (0.49)	0.99
Creatinine mg/dL, mean (SD)	0.85 (0.14)	0.85 (0.45)	0.14
Hemoglobin g/dL, mean (SD)	14 (1.9)	14.3 (1.7)	0.51
Platelets, ×1000/μL, mean (SD)	100 (54)	128 (71)	0.04
HCV RNA ×10^6 IU/mL, mean (SD)	1.79 (1.33)	1.8 (3.45)	0.03

BMI, body mass index; SD, standard deviation; HBV, hepatitis B virus; HBsAg+, hepatitis B surface antigen; HIV, human immunodeficiency virus; HCC, hepatocellular carcinoma; IFN, interferon; DAA, direct-acting antivirals; ALT, alanine transaminase; HCV RNA, ribonucleic acid of hepatitis C virus.

Table 7. Treatment effectiveness in subpopulations.

	Females, n = 66	Males, n = 170	p
SVR ITT	97% (64/66)	85.3% (145/170)	0.01
SVR PP	97% (64/66)	87.3% (145/166)	0.03
	HCV RNA < 1,000,000, n = 131	HCV RNA ≥ 1,000,000, n = 105	
SVR ITT	93.1% (122/131)	82.9% (87/105)	0.02
SVR PP	95.3% (122/128)	83.7% (87/104)	0.004
	Treatment-experienced, n = 66	Treatment-naive, n = 170	
SVR ITT	81.8% (54/66)	91.2% (155/170)	0.07
SVR PP	85.7% (54/63)	91.7% (155/169)	0.22
	DAA-experienced, n = 49	Treatment-naive, n = 170	
SVR ITT	77.5% (38/49)	91.2% (155/170)	0.02
SVR PP	80.9% (38/47)	91.7% (155/169)	0.06
	BMI < 30, n = 161	BMI ≥ 30, n = 64	
SVR ITT	88.2% (142/161)	92.2% (59/64)	0.48
SVR PP	89.9% (142/158)	92.2% (59/64)	0.80

SVR, sustained virologic response; ITT, intent to treat; PP, per protocol; HCV RNA, ribonucleic acid of hepatitis C virus; IFN, interferon; DAA, direct-acting antivirals; SOF, sofosbuvir; BMI, body mass index; The bold represent the same level as gender.

Table 8. Baseline factors associated with SVR based on the logistic regression model.

	Estimate of β	SE	t-Stat	p Value
(Intercept)			550.76	<0.001
Gender (male)	−0.16	0.07	−2.47	0.01
Baseline ascites (no)	0.17	0.07	2.43	0.03
Previous decompensation (no)	0.04	0.07	0.59	0.55
Response to previous therapy (non-response)	0.04	0.09	0.51	0.61
Response to previous therapy (naive)	0.11	0.09	1.22	0.22
Bilirubin	0.03	0.07	0.34	0.73
Platelets	0.05	0.07	0.71	0.48
HCV RNA	0.02	0.06	0.34	0.73

HCV RNA, ribonucleic acid of hepatitis C virus.

The majority of patients completed the treatment course according to schedule, 98.2% in GLE/PIB and 93% in SOF/VEL ± RBV, 6.2% of patients receiving RBV experienced dose modification, three patients discontinued treatment, two due to adverse events (AE), and one by his own decision. A similar proportion of patients in both subpopulations reported at least one AE, with the most common pruritus/skin changes in the course of GLE/PIB treatment and weakness/fatigue during SOF/VEL ± RBV therapy (Table 9).

Table 9. Safety of GLE/PIB and SOF/VEL ± RBV in GT3 infected patients with liver cirrhosis.

Parameter	GLE/PIB n = 107	SOF/VEL ± RBV n = 129	p
Treatment course, n (%)			
according to schedule	105 (98.2)	120 (93)	0.12
modified RBV dosage	Na	8 (6.2)	Na
therapy discontinuation	2 (1.8)	1 (0.8) *	0.59
Patients with at least one AE	24 (22.4)	28 (21.7)	1.00
Most common AEs			
weakness/fatigue	7 (6.5)	12 (9.3)	0.48
gastrointestinal symptoms	4 (3.7)	7 (5.4)	0.76
pruritus/skin changes	8 (7.5)	2 (1.6)	0.05
anemia	0	9 (7)	0.004

Table 9. Cont.

Parameter	GLE/PIB n = 107	SOF/VEL ± RBV n = 129	p
Death	0	0	na
Other serious adverse events	0	3 (2.3) **	0.25
AEs leading to treatment discontinuation	2 (1.8) ***	0	0.20
AEs of particular interest			
ascites	2 (1.8)	2 (1.6)	1.00
hepatic encephalopathy	0	1 (0.8)	1.00
gastrointestinal bleeding	0	2 (1.6)	0.50

* patient's decision; ** hepatic decompensation, HCC, pneumonia; *** worsening of depression, exacerbation of heart failure; GLE, glecaprevir; PIB, pibrentasvir; SOF, sofosbuvir; VEL, velpatasvir; RBV, ribavirin; AE, adverse event.

Three serious AE in patients treated with SOF/VEL + RBV, but not related to this regimen, were documented. In addition, seven AEs of particular interest related to the deterioration of the liver function were reported, including ascites in 4 patients, gastrointestinal bleeding in 2 individuals, and hepatic encephalopathy in one person.

4. Discussion

After more than four years elapsed since the registration of the highly potent pangenotypic regimens, the published data from real-world experience (RWE) studies on the use of these medications in GT3 infected patients with liver cirrhosis are still limited, and most of them included a small number of patients.

The single tablet SOF/VEL combination was the first available highly effective option registered for patients with CHC regardless of the HCV genotype, the history of previous therapy, and liver fibrosis. For those with GT3 infection and liver cirrhosis, a 12-week treatment duration was approved based on the results of clinical trials demonstrating cure rates of 91–93%, which is comparable to 93% reported in our analysis [15–17]. The better efficacy of 97.5% was achieved in RWE analysis performed by Mangia et al. among 205 Italian GT3 infected patients with liver cirrhosis despite the higher percentage of CP B patients compared to our cohort [18]. However, it should be noted that no DAA-experienced patients were included in the study in contrast to our analysis. The population treated with SOF/VEL in 16 clinical practice cohorts worldwide comprising also DAA-experienced individuals except NS5A-containing regimens achieved an SVR of 93% (332/356) [19]. On the other hand, the cure rate following the SOF/VEL option reported among the RWE cohort of American Veterans, including previously untreated and those who received both IFN- and DAA-based regimens, was 86.5%, lower compared to our result [20].

Even lower efficacy of 79% was achieved in the current analysis in patients treated with SOF/VEL and RBV. It should be noted that the addition of RBV is an option to consider in compensated cirrhotics infected with GT3, whereas it is recommended in the case of decompensated individuals for whom the SOF/VEL is the only registered DAA pangenotypic regimen [21]. The differences in baseline characteristics of patients with a significantly higher number of those with more severe liver disease and the higher rate of treatment-experienced ones among individuals receiving therapy with RBV seem to be the difference of great importance that affects the effectiveness of the treatment with SOF/VEL regimen. Our findings on lower SVR with the SOF/VEL + RBV regimen contradict the results of clinical trials with 96% cure rates, but both studies included only IFN-based treatment-experienced individuals [16,17].

The SVR rate of 95.5% (192/201) was reported for SOF/VEL + RBV option in analysis from multinational RWE presented by Fagiuoli et al., but the range was between 88% and 100% [19]. Mangia et al. documented a 90.5% cure rate with SOF/VEL + RBV regimen in the RWE population, but only ten GT3 infected patients with liver cirrhosis were included [22]. The efficacy of 88% was demonstrated in a real-life population consisted of 34 patients, including 31 treatment-experienced with both IFN- and DAA-based except

NS5A-containing regimens [23]. The much more numerous RWE cohort comprising 267 cirrhotic American Veterans treated with SOF/VEL + RBV analyzed by Belperio et al., including NS5A-experienced individuals, responded in 84.5% [20]. Since the failure of prior antiviral therapy, especially DAA containing antiviral therapy, is well recognized as a negative predictor of SVR, the low efficacy documented in our analysis may be influenced by a high percentage of nonresponders in the SOF/VEL + RBV arm, 26/58 (45%), with of whom 21 were treated with DAA [24]. Nine of them received a longer therapy duration 24 weeks, seven responded to treatment, and one was lost to follow-up, giving an 87.5% SVR rate in PP analysis. According to the label, the longer treatment course of SOF/VEL + RBV may be considered in patients who have failed therapy with an NS5A-containing regimen based on analysis from phase 2 and 3 clinical trials. However, there are no clinical data to support this recommendation [21,25]. Therefore further studies are needed to clarify the need for ribavirin in the treatment of decompensated genotype 3 infected cirrhotics who failed previous DAA-based therapy. In the current analysis, six of eight NS5A-experienced patients were treated with SOF/VEL + RBV; three of them failed to achieve an SVR, two with 12-week and another with a 24-week regimen. The remaining two NS5A-experienced patients underwent successful treatment with a 16-week GLE/PIB regimen; however, the numbers are too small to draw conclusions.

The dual therapy of GLE/PIB was approved for GT3 infected patients with compensated liver cirrhosis, and initially, a 12-week option was recommended for treatment-naïve and a 16-week regimen for treatment-experienced individuals based on the results from the clinical trials [26]. With the update of the label made upon the findings from the EXPEDITION-8 trial treatment-naïve, GT3 infected cirrhotics received the possibility to shorten the therapy length to 8 weeks without losing efficacy [27]. In our analysis, the majority of treatment-naïve patients were assigned to a 12-week regimen with an efficacy rate of 97%, while treatment-experienced individuals responded in 95% to 16-week therapy, which is comparable to 98% and 96% SVR rates documented in SURVEYOR-II part 3 study [28]. The data pooled from five phase 2 and 3 clinical trials, including a total of 120 patients with compensated liver cirrhosis, documented a 97% efficacy rate in treatment-naïve following 12-week therapy and 94% as a result of 16-week regimen in treatment-experienced patients [29]. A higher cure rate of 100% was reported in 12 cirrhotic patients from the German Hepatitis-C Registry receiving GLE/PIB, and among Italian cirrhotics treated for 12 or 16 weeks depending on the history of previous treatment, but no precise information on the number of patients, in this case, was added [30,31]. A lower SVR of 83% was demonstrated in 6 treatment-naïve cirrhotic GT3 infected individuals by Toyoda et al. [32]. Very limited RWE data based on small numbers of patients are available for treatment-naïve GT3 infected patients with liver cirrhosis treated with GLE/PIB for 8 weeks. The first published paper from the USA reported a 100% response rate in a group of 4 patients [33]. The same effectiveness was documented by Lampertico et al. following the 8-week GLE/PIB treatment duration in 19 cirrhotic patients with GT3 infection from seven small RWE studies included in the summary analysis [34,35]. A much lower SVR of 72% in PP analysis was demonstrated in nine GT3 infected cirrhotics in our previous study from the EpiTer-2 database, but it was due to a small subset of patients [36]. In the current study, 16 patients treated for 8 weeks achieved SVR, which gives an unsatisfactory rate of 84% in PP analysis, lower than demonstrated for a 12-week regimen with statistical significance for ITT analysis (80% vs. 95.4%, $p = 0.05$), however, it should be noted that a number of patients on 8-week regimen was still low. Further investigations in a large population of GT3 infected cirrhotics are needed to assess the real-world efficacy of an 8-week GLE/PIB regimen. According to label glecaprevir as a protease inhibitor included in the glecaprevir/pibrentasvir regimen is not recommended in moderate hepatic impairment (Child-Pugh B), and is contraindicated in Child-Pugh C patients only. Our study did not include patients with Child-Pugh C and only 4.7% of those treated with glecaprevir/pibrentasvir were classified as Child-Pugh B. The decision to use a protease inhibitor (glecaprevir) in a patient with Child-Pugh B was made by the treating physician.

According to the best of our knowledge, only two available studies made a direct comparison between different pangenotypic regimens in GT3 infected patients, including those with compensated liver cirrhosis. One of them is the analysis performed among 76 Spanish patients with GT3 infection, of whom 12 were diagnosed as cirrhotics, nine were treated with SOF/VEL, including three receiving RBV additionally, and three were assigned to GLE/PIB. The reported efficacy rates were 89% for SOF/VEL ± RBV (8/9) regimen and 67% (2/3) for GLE/PIB option [37]. The second available RWE study comparing SOF/VEL ± RBV, GLE/PIB, and SOF/DCV regimens in GT3 infected patients was made by Soria et al. in a multicentre cohort of Italian patients [38]. Ninety-nine of 2082 individuals included in the study had liver cirrhosis, and despite the difference in SVR rates with 100% in 21 patients treated with GLE/PIB and 93.6% among 78 those receiving SOF/VEL ± RBV regimen, no statistical significance was demonstrated. The comparative analysis concerning demographic, clinical, and laboratory variables between two cirrhotic subpopulations was not provided since the primary comparison was performed among GT3 patients regardless of the liver fibrosis.

No specific safety issues were observed during the treatment course, and we confirmed comparable tolerability across regimens with only a higher rate of RBV-related anemia in SOF/VEL ± RBV. Our findings are in line with the results of clinical trials and RWE studies [15–18].

The several limitations of the current study related to its real-world nature and retrospective observational design could be identified. Firstly, some clinical data might have been under-reported, including mild adverse events, the prevalence of comorbidities, and concomitant medications usage. No drug monitoring during the therapy hampers the assessment of compliance and its impact on the treatment efficacy. Electronic data capture might result in possible data entry errors. No resistance-associated substitutions (RAS) in previously DAA-nonresponders were tested at baseline. The choice of a therapeutic regimen in all patients was based on the treating physician's decision regarding recommendations and regulations. However, according to the most recent EASL guidelines, if resistance testing is available and performed, only DAA-experienced patients with the NS5A Y93H RAS at baseline should be treated with SOF/VEL plus RBV, whereas those without should receive SOF/VEL alone, so we assumed that this factor did not affect efficacy reported in our analysis, no NS5A-experienced patient was treated with SOL/VEL [11,39]. Noteworthy, the other regimen prescribed in GT3 infected patients with the presence of Y93H RAS is the combination of SOF/VEL and protease inhibitor voxilaprevir is not recommended in decompensated cirrhotics; moreover, it was not available in Poland within a reimbursed therapeutic program in the analyzed period. Furthermore, finally, since the possibility for a shorter 8-weeks treatment course with GLE/PIB in treatment-naïve GT3 infected patients with liver cirrhosis has emerged very recently, the subset of this population in our analysis is relatively small. However, the study's major strength is collecting data from the real-world, heterogeneous population representative of routine practice. Moreover, in this study, we included a high number of patients with a low rate of those lost to follow-up (<2%).

5. Conclusions

In summary, we confirmed the overall high effectiveness and safety of pangenotypic regimens in the real-world setting of cirrhotics with chronic genotype 3 HCV infection. The highest effectiveness was achieved in those treated with the GLE/PIB regimen, but it was suboptimal if therapy was carried out for 8 weeks. The addition of ribavirin to the SOF/VEL regimen was associated with significantly decreased effectiveness. However, it was related to hepatic decompensation at baseline and failure of previous DAA-based therapy, which are currently indications for ribavirin coadministration. Further studies are needed to clarify the real need for ribavirin in such a difficult-to-treat population of patients treated with SOF/VEL.

Author Contributions: Conceptualization—D.Z.-M., R.F., methodology—D.Z.-M., R.F., formal analysis—D.Z.-M., J.J., investigation—D.Z.-M., validation—R.F., writing—original draft preparation—D.Z.-M., writing—review and editing—R.F., supervision—R.F., project administration—R.F., data collection—D.Z.-M., J.J., A.P.-K., E.J., D.D., M.P., W.H., W.M., B.L., J.J.-L., K.S., A.P., H.B., J.K., P.S., B.S.-S., J.C., Ł.S., M.T.-Z., K.T., M.S., B.D., R.K., J.B.-W., Ł.L., R.F. All authors have read and agreed to the published version of the manuscript.

Funding: This research received no external funding.

Institutional Review Board Statement: This observational study was conducted in a real-world setting with approved drugs. Patients were not exposed to any experimental interventions nor did the study intervene with the clinical management of the patient. The study only collected information from patient medical records. The analysis included routine examinations and tests performed in patients treated within the therapeutic program of the National Health Fund. The data were originally collected to assess treatment efficacy and safety in individual patients, not for scientific purposes. Hence, the treating physicians did not obtain approval from the ethics committee. According to local law (Pharmaceutical Law of 6 September 2001, art. 37al), non-interventional studies do not require ethics committee approval.

Informed Consent Statement: Patient consent was waived due to the retrospective design of the study.

Data Availability Statement: Data supporting reported results can be provided upon request from the corresponding author.

Acknowledgments: The authors wish to thank Tadeusz Łapiński, who helped in data collection but who had sadly passed away before the manuscript submission.

Conflicts of Interest: The authors declare no conflict of interest.

References

1. World Health Organization. *Global Health Sector Strategy on Viral Hepatitis 2016–2021*; World Health Organization: Geneva, Switzerland, 2016. Available online: http://apps.who.int/iris/bitstream/10665/246177/1/WHO-HIV-2016.06-eng.pdf?ua=1 (accessed on 13 June 2021).
2. Westbrook, R.H.; Dusheiko, G. Natural history of hepatitis C. *J. Hepatol.* **2014**, *61* (Suppl. 1), S58–S68. [CrossRef]
3. Kanwal, F.; Kramer, J.R.; Ilyas, J.; Duan, Z.; El-Serag, H.B. HCV genotype 3 is associated with an increased risk of cirrhosis and hepatocellular cancer in a national sample of U.S. Veterans with HCV. *Hepatology* **2014**, *60*, 98–105. [CrossRef]
4. Nkontchou, G.; Ziol, M.; Aout, M.; Lhabadie, M.; Baazia, Y.; Mahmoudi, A.; Roulot, D.; Ganne-Carrie, N.; Grando-Lemaire, V.; Trinchet, J.C.; et al. HCV genotype 3 is associated with a higher hepatocellular carcinoma incidence in patients with ongoing viral C cirrhosis. *J. Viral. Hepat.* **2011**, *18*, e516–e522. [CrossRef]
5. Messina, J.P.; Humphreys, I.; Flaxman, A.; Brown, A.; Cooke, G.S.; Pybus, O.G.; Barnes, E. Global distribution and prevalence of hepatitis C virus genotypes. *Hepatology* **2015**, *61*, 77–87. [CrossRef]
6. Flisiak, R.; Pogorzelska, J.; Berak, H.; Horban, A.; Orłowska, I.; Simon, K.; Tuchendler, E.; Madej, G.; Piekarska, A.; Jabłkowski, M.; et al. Prevalence of HCV genotypes in Poland—The EpiTer study. *Clin. Exp. Hepatol* **2016**, *2*, 144–148. [CrossRef]
7. Flisiak, R.; Pogorzelska, J.; Berak, H.; Horban, A.; Orłowska, I.; Simon, K.; Tuchendler, E.; Madej, G.; Piekarska, A.; Jabłkowski, M.; et al. Efficacy of HCV treatment in Poland at the turn of the interferon era—The EpiTer study. *Clin. Exp. Hepatol.* **2016**, *2*, 138–143. [CrossRef]
8. Foster, G.R.; Pianko, S.; Brown, A.; Forton, D.; Nahass, R.G.; George, J.; Barnes, E.; Brainard, D.M.; Massetto, B.; Lin, M.; et al. Efficacy of sofosbuvir plus ribavirin with or without peginterferon-alfa in patients with hepatitis C virus genotype 3 infection and treatment-experienced patients with cirrhosis and hepatitis C virus genotype 2 infection. *Gastroenterology* **2015**, *149*, 1462–1470. [CrossRef] [PubMed]
9. Poordad, F.; Shiffman, M.L.; Ghesquiere, W.; Wong, A.; Huhn, G.D.; Wong, F.; Ramji, A.; Shafran, S.D.; McPhee, F.; Yang, R.; et al. Daclatasvir and sofosbuvir with ribavirin for 24 wk in chronic hepatitis C genotype-3-infected patients with cirrhosis: A Phase III study (ALLY-3C). *Antivir. Ther.* **2019**, *24*, 35–44. [CrossRef] [PubMed]
10. Zarębska-Michaluk, D.; Flisiak, R.; Jaroszewicz, J.; Janczewska, E.; Czauż-Andrzejuk, A.; Berak, H.; Horban, A.; Staniaszek, A.; Gietka, A.; Tudrujek, M.; et al. Is Interferon-Based Treatment of Viral Hepatitis C Genotype 3 Infection Still of Value in the Era of Direct-Acting Antivirals? *J. Interferon Cytokine Res.* **2018**, *38*, 93–100. [CrossRef] [PubMed]
11. European Association for the Study of the Liver. Clinical Practice Guidelines Panel: Chair, EASL Governing Board representative, Panel members. EASL recommendations on treatment of hepatitis C: Final update of the series. *J. Hepatol.* **2020**, *73*, 1170–1218. [CrossRef]

12. Ghany, M.G.; Morgan, T.R.; AASLD-IDSA Hepatitis C Guidance Panel. Hepatitis C Guidance 2019 Update: American Association for the Study of Liver Diseases-Infectious Diseases Society of America Recommendations for Testing, Managing, and Treating Hepatitis C Virus Infection. *Hepatology* **2020**, *71*, 686–721. [CrossRef]
13. Halota, W.; Flisiak, R.; Juszczyk, J.; Małkowski, P.; Pawłowska, M.; Simon, K.; Tomasiewicz, K. Recommendations of the Polish Group of Experts for HCV for the treatment of hepatitis C in 2020. *Clin. Exp. Hepatol.* **2020**, *6*, 163–169. [CrossRef]
14. Zarębska-Michaluk, D. Genotype 3-hepatitis C virus' last line of defense. *World J. Gastroenterol.* **2021**, *27*, 1006–1021. [CrossRef]
15. Foster, G.R.; Afdhal, N.; Roberts, S.K.; Bräu, N.; Gane, E.J.; Pianko, S.; Lawitz, E.; Thompson, A.; Shiffman, M.L.; Cooper, C.; et al. Sofosbuvir and Velpatasvir for HCV Genotype 2 and 3 Infection. *N. Engl. J. Med.* **2015**, *373*, 2608–2617. [CrossRef]
16. Pianko, S.; Flamm, S.L.; Shiffman, M.L.; Kumar, S.; Strasser, S.I.; Dore, G.J.; McNally, J.; Brainard, D.M.; Han, L.; Doehle, B.; et al. Sofosbuvir Plus Velpatasvir Combination Therapy for Treatment-Experienced Patients With Genotype 1 or 3 Hepatitis C Virus Infection: A Randomized Trial. *Ann. Intern. Med.* **2015**, *163*, 809–817. [CrossRef]
17. Esteban, R.; Pineda, J.A.; Calleja, J.L.; Casado, M.; Rodríguez, M.; Turnes, J.; Morano Amado, L.E.; Morillas, R.M.; Forns, X.; Pascasio Acevedo, J.M.; et al. Efficacy of Sofosbuvir and Velpatasvir, With and Without Ribavirin, in Patients With Hepatitis C Virus Genotype 3 Infection and Cirrhosis. *Gastroenterology* **2018**, *155*, 1120–1127. [CrossRef] [PubMed]
18. Mangia, A.; Cenderello, G.; Copetti, M.; Verucchi, G.; Piazzolla, V.; Lorusso, C.; Santoro, R.; Squillante, M.M.; Orlandini, A.; Minisini, R.; et al. SVR12 Higher than 97% in GT3 Cirrhotic Patients with Evidence of Portal Hypertension Treated with SOF/VEL without Ribavirin: A Nation-Wide Cohort Study. *Cells* **2019**, *8*, 313. [CrossRef] [PubMed]
19. Fagiuoli, S.; Agarwal, K.; Mangia, A.; Shafran, S.D.; Wedemeyer, H.; Terrault, N.; Feld, J.J.; Turnes, J.; Buggish, P.; Ciancio, A.; et al. Effectiveness of Sofosbuvir/Velpatasvir for 12 weeks in HCV genotype 3 patients with compensated cirrhosis in clinical practice cohorts from around the world. *Hepatology* **2018**, *68* (Suppl. 1), 360A–361A.
20. Belperio, P.S.; Shahoumian, T.A.; Loomis, T.P.; Mole, L.A.; Backus, L.I. Real-world effectiveness of daclatasvir plus sofosbuvir and velpatasvir/sofosbuvir in hepatitis C genotype 2 and 3. *J. Hepatol.* **2019**, *70*, 15–23. [CrossRef] [PubMed]
21. Epclusa Summary of Product Characteristics. 2020. Available online: https://www.ema.europa.eu/en/medicines/human/EPAR/epclusa#product-information-section (accessed on 13 June 2021).
22. Mangia, A.; Losappio, R.; Cenderello, G.; Potenza, D.; Mazzola, M.; De Stefano, G.; Terreni, N.; Copetti, M.; Minerva, N.; Piazzola, V.; et al. Real life rates of sustained virological response (SVR) and predictors of relapse following DAA treatment in genotype 3 (GT3) patients with advanced fibrosis/cirrhosis. *PLoS ONE* **2018**, *13*, e0200568. [CrossRef] [PubMed]
23. Mushtaq, S.; Akhter, T.S.; Khan, A.; Sohail, A.; Khan, A.; Manzoor, S. Efficacy and Safety of Generic Sofosbuvir Plus Daclatasvir and Sofosbuvir/Velpatasvir in HCV Genotype 3-Infected Patients: Real-World Outcomes from Pakistan. *Front. Pharmacol.* **2020**, *11*, 550205. [CrossRef] [PubMed]
24. Llerena, S.; Cabezas, J.; Cuadrado, A.; Manuel Olmos, J.; González, M.; García, F.; Cobo, C.; Crespo, J. Rescue Therapy for Genotype-3 DAA Non-responders, Almost all Done. *Ann. Hepatol.* **2019**, *18*, 236–239. [CrossRef] [PubMed]
25. Gane, E.J.; Shiffman, M.L.; Etzkorn, K.; Morelli, G.; Stedman, C.A.M.; Davis, M.N.; Hinestrosa, F.; Dvory-Sobol, H.; Huang, K.C.; Osinusi, A.; et al. Sofosbuvir-velpatasvir with ribavirin for 24 weeks in hepatitis C virus patients previously treated with a direct-acting antiviral regimen. *Hepatology* **2017**, *66*, 1083–1089. [CrossRef]
26. European Medicines Agency. EMA/332999/2020. *Maviret: Procedural Steps Taken and Scientific Information after the Authorization.* Available online: https://www.ema.europa.eu/en/documents/procedural-steps-after/maviret-epar-procedural-steps-taken-scientific-information-after-authorisation_en.pdf (accessed on 13 June 2021).
27. Brown, R.S., Jr.; Buti, M.; Rodrigues, L.; Chulanov, V.; Chuang, W.L.; Aguilar, H.; Horváth, G.; Zuckerman, E.; Carrion, B.R.; Rodriguez-Perez, F.; et al. Glecaprevir/pibrentasvir for 8 wk in treatment-naïve patients with chronic HCV genotypes 1-6 and compensated cirrhosis: The EXPEDITION-8 trial. *J. Hepatol.* **2020**, *72*, 441–449. [CrossRef]
28. Wyles, D.; Poordad, F.; Wang, S.; Alric, L.; Felizarta, F.; Kwo, P.Y.; Maliakkal, B.; Agarwal, K.; Hassanein, T.; Weilert, F.; et al. Glecaprevir/pibrentasvir for hepatitis C virus genotype 3 patients with cirrhosis and/or prior treatment experience: A partially randomized phase 3 clinical trial. *Hepatology* **2018**, *67*, 514–523. [CrossRef] [PubMed]
29. Flamm, S.; Mutimer, D.; Asatryan, A.; Wang, S.; Rockstroh, J.; Horsmans, Y.; Kwo, P.Y.; Weiland, O.; Villa, E.; Heo, J.; et al. Glecaprevir/Pibrentasvir in patients with chronic HCV genotype 3 infection: An integrated phase 2/3 analysis. *J. Viral. Hepat.* **2019**, *26*, 337–349. [CrossRef] [PubMed]
30. Berg, T.; Naumann, U.; Stoehr, A.; Sick, C.; John, C.; Teuber, G.; Schiffelholz, W.; Mauss, S.; Lohmann, K.; König, B.; et al. Real-world effectiveness and safety of glecaprevir/pibrentasvir for the treatment of chronic hepatitis C infection: Data from the German Hepatitis C-Registry. *Aliment. Pharmacol. Ther.* **2019**, *49*, 1052–1059. [CrossRef]
31. D'Ambrosio, R.; Pasulo, L.; Puoti, M.; Vinci, M.; Schiavini, M.; Lazzaroni, S.; Soria, A.; Gatti, F.; Menzaghi, B.; Aghemo, A.; et al. NAVIGATORE-Lombardia Study Group. Real-world effectiveness and safety of glecaprevir/pibrentasvir in 723 patients with chronic hepatitis C. *J. Hepatol.* **2019**, *70*, 379–387. [CrossRef]
32. Toyoda, H.; Atsukawa, M.; Watanabe, T.; Nakamuta, M.; Uojima, H.; Nozaki, A.; Takaguchi, K.; Fujioka, S.; Iio, E.; Shima, T.; et al. Real-world experience of 12-week direct-acting antiviral regimen of glecaprevir and pibrentasvir in patients with chronic hepatitis C virus infection. *J. Gastroenterol. Hepatol.* **2020**, *35*, 855–861. [CrossRef]
33. Flamm, S.L.; Kort, J.; Marx, S.E.; Strezewski, J.; Dylla, D.E.; Bacon, B.; Curry, M.P.; Tsai, N.; Wick, N. Effectiveness of 8-Week Glecaprevir/Pibrentasvir for Treatment-Naïve, Compensated Cirrhotic Patients with Chronic Hepatitis C Infection. *Adv. Ther.* **2020**, *37*, 2267–2274. [CrossRef]

34. Lampertico, P.; Mauss, S.; Persico, M.; Barclay, S.T.; Marx, S.; Lohmann, K.; Bondin, M.; Zhang, Z.; Marra, F.; Belperio, P.S.; et al. Real-World Clinical Practice Use of 8-Week Glecaprevir/Pibrentasvir in Treatment-Naïve Patients with Compensated Cirrhosis. *Adv. Ther.* **2020**, *37*, 4033–4042. [CrossRef] [PubMed]
35. Belperio, P.; Shahoumian, T.; Loomis, T.; Mole, L.; Backus, L. Real-world effectiveness of glecaprevir/pibrentasvir in 1,941 patients with hepatitis C genotypes 1 through 4. *Hepatology* **2018**, *68*, 417A–418A.
36. Zarębska-Michaluk, D.; Jaroszewicz, J.; Pabjan, P.; Łapiński, T.W.; Mazur, W.; Krygier, R.; Dybowska, D.; Halota, W.; Pawłowska, M.; Janczewska, E.; et al. Is an 8-week regimen of glecaprevir/pibrentasvir sufficient for all hepatitis C virus infected patients in the real-world experience? *J. Gastroenterol. Hepatol.* **2020**. [CrossRef]
37. Margusino-Framiñán, L.; Cid-Silva, P.; Rotea-Salvo, S.; Mena-de-Cea, Á.; Suárez-López, F.; Vázquez-Rodríguez, P.; Delgado-Blanco, M.; Sanclaudio-Luhia, A.I.; Martín-Herranz, I.; Castro-Iglesias, Á. Effectiveness and safety of sofosbuvir/velpatasvir ± ribavirin vs. glecaprevir/pibrentasvir in genotype 3 hepatitis C virus infected patients. *Eur. J. Hosp. Pharm.* **2020**, *27*, e41–e47. [CrossRef] [PubMed]
38. Soria, A.; Fava, M.; Bernasconi, D.P.; Lapadula, G.; Colella, E.; Valsecchi, M.G.; Migliorino, G.M.; D'Ambrosio, R.; Landonio, S.; Schiavini, M.; et al. Comparison of three therapeutic regimens for genotype-3 hepatitis C virus infection in a large real-life multicentre cohort. *Liver Int.* **2020**, *40*, 769–777. [CrossRef]
39. Sarrazin, C. Treatment failure with DAA therapy: Importance of resistance. *J. Hepatol.* **2021**. [CrossRef] [PubMed]

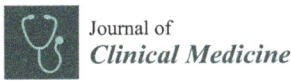

Article

Real-Life Experience with Ledipasvir/Sofosbuvir for the Treatment of Chronic Hepatitis C Virus Infection with Genotypes 1 and 4 in Children Aged 12 to 17 Years—Results of the POLAC Project

Maria Pokorska-Śpiewak [1,2,*], Anna Dobrzeniecka [2], Małgorzata Aniszewska [1,2] and Magdalena Marczyńska [1,2]

[1] Department of Children's Infectious Diseases, Regional Hospital of Infectious Diseases in Warsaw, Medical University of Warsaw, Wolska Str. 37, 01-201 Warsaw, Poland; malgorzata.aniszewska@wum.edu.pl (M.A.); magdalena.marczynska@wum.edu.pl (M.M.)
[2] Department of Pediatric Infectious Diseases, Regional Hospital of Infectious Diseases in Warsaw, 01-201 Warsaw, Poland; adobrzeniecka@zakazny.pl
* Correspondence: mpspiewak@gmail.com; Tel.: +48-22-33-55-250; Fax: +48-22-33-55-379

Citation: Pokorska-Śpiewak, M.; Dobrzeniecka, A.; Aniszewska, M.; Marczyńska, M. Real-Life Experience with Ledipasvir/Sofosbuvir for the Treatment of Chronic Hepatitis C Virus Infection with Genotypes 1 and 4 in Children Aged 12 to 17 Years—Results of the POLAC Project. *J. Clin. Med.* **2021**, *10*, 4176. https://doi.org/10.3390/jcm10184176

Academic Editors: Maria Carla Liberto and Nadia Marascio

Received: 12 August 2021
Accepted: 14 September 2021
Published: 15 September 2021

Publisher's Note: MDPI stays neutral with regard to jurisdictional claims in published maps and institutional affiliations.

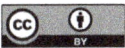

Copyright: © 2021 by the authors. Licensee MDPI, Basel, Switzerland. This article is an open access article distributed under the terms and conditions of the Creative Commons Attribution (CC BY) license (https://creativecommons.org/licenses/by/4.0/).

Abstract: Background: Available real-world data on the efficacy and safety of ledipasvir/sofosbuvir (LDV/SOF) in pediatric patients are limited. In this prospective, open-label, single-center study, we aimed to present our real-life experience with a fixed dose of LDV/SOF (90/400 mg) for the treatment of chronic hepatitis C (CHC) genotypes 1 and 4 in children aged 12 to 17 years. Methods: We analyzed intention-to-treat (ITT) and per-protocol (PP) rates of sustained virological response (SVR), defined as undetectable HCV viral load at posttreatment week 12, in 37 participants treated with LDV/SOF according to the HCV genotype, baseline liver fibrosis, duration of treatment, and experience of the previous ineffective antiviral treatment. There were 32 patients infected with genotype 1 and 5 with genotype 4. Fourteen (38%) participants were treatment-experienced, two were coinfected with HIV, and three were cirrhotic. Two patients qualified for 24 weeks of therapy, and the remaining 35 received 12 weeks of LDV/SOF treatment. Results: The overall ITT SVR12 rate was 36/37 (97%). One patient was lost to follow-up after week 4 of therapy when his HCV RNA was undetectable. All 36 patients who completed the full protocol achieved SVR (36/36, 100%). PP analyses of SVR12 rates according to the HCV genotype, baseline liver fibrosis, duration of the treatment, and previous ineffective treatment were all 100%. A significant decrease in aminotransferase serum levels was observed in the subsequent weeks of the treatment and at SVR assessment compared to baseline. No serious adverse events were reported. Conclusions: The results of this study confirm previous observations of a suitable efficacy and safety profile of LDV/SOF for the treatment of CHC genotypes 1 and 4 in adolescents.

Keywords: children; hepatitis C; ledipasvir/sofosbuvir; real-life; sustained virological response

1. Background

It is estimated that over 3.25 million (95% confidence interval 2.07–3.90) children are infected with hepatitis C virus (HCV) globally, which corresponds to a prevalence of 0.13% (0.08–0.16) [1]. Among them, 3500 (2600–4200) subjects are considered to be living in Poland, which makes the HCV prevalence 0.05 (0.04–0.06) [1]. However, according to the data published by the National Institute of Public Health, Warsaw, Poland, between 2010 and 2019, only 545 cases of hepatitis C were reported in patients aged 0–19 years, which suggests that most cases of HCV-infected children remain undiagnosed [2]. Chronic hepatitis C (CHC) in children is usually considered a mild disease with only a slow progression of liver disease. However, recent studies reported a significant proportion of pediatric patients who develop significant fibrosis or even cirrhosis as a result of early infection with HCV [3–5]. In addition, Younossi et al. [6] showed that HCV infection in adolescents may be associated with decreased health-related quality of life, poor social functioning, and a reduction in intelligence and memory testing. To prevent these consequences of CHC, early anti-HCV treatment should be implemented. New, extremely effective, and safe interferon-free therapies based on direct-acting antivirals (DAAs) have significantly changed the natural history of CHC, and they have provided a chance for HCV eradication [7]. The first DAA, ledipasvir/sofosbuvir (LDV/SOF), was approved for use in children aged 12–17 years by the European Medical Agency (EMA), Amsterdam, The Netherlands, and U.S. Food and Drug Administration (FDA), Silver Spring, MD, US, in 2017 [8]. Since 2019, LDV/SOF has been used in children aged at least 3 years [9,10]. However, due to the prohibitive prices of DAAs, only a few countries have included recommendations for the treatment of pediatric patients infected with HCV in their national policies and strategies [11,12]. Thus, only a small proportion of children and adolescents with CHC have been treated, mainly during clinical trials. As a result, available real-world data on the efficacy and safety of LDV/SOF in pediatric patients are limited [13,14]. Thus, in this prospective, single-arm, observational, open-label single-center study, we aimed to present our real-life experience with LDV/SOF for the treatment of CHC in children aged 12 to 17 years infected with HCV genotypes 1 and 4.

2. Materials and Methods

In Poland, patients below 18 years of age are not included in the national therapeutic programs for CHC. However, courtesy of a donation of LDV/SOF by the pharmaceutical company in August 2019, our single tertiary health care pediatric infectious disease department launched the real-life therapeutic program 'Treatment of Polish Adolescents with Chronic Hepatitis C Using Direct Acting Antivirals (POLAC project)'. In this project, we qualified consecutive patients aged 12–17 years (weighing at least 35 kg) infected with genotype 1 and 4 HCV for therapy with LDV/SOF (fixed-dose tablet of 90/400 mg). CHC was diagnosed in subjects with over a 6-month duration of disease confirmed with positive nucleic acid testing, HCV RNA, using quantitative real-time polymerase chain reaction (RT-PCR) (Abbott RealTime HCV, Abbott Laboratories, Abbott Park, Illinois, USA; measurement linearity range 12–1.0 $\times$ 10^8 IU/mL). Patients were eligible for the treatment regardless of the extent of liver fibrosis or previous ineffective treatment. The duration of treatment was established according to the recommendations of the European Society of Pediatric Gastroenterology, Hepatology and Nutrition (ESPGHAN), Geneva, Switzerland: patients received 12 weeks of therapy unless they were infected with HCV genotype 1 with a history of previous ineffective interferon-based treatment and presented with cirrhosis. This specific group of patients was treated for 24 weeks [15]. Before starting the treatment, the possibility of drug interactions between LDV/SOF and other medicines received by the patient was excluded using the online HEP Drug Interactions Checker provided by the University of Liverpool (www.hep-druginteractions.org).

2.1. Treatment Monitoring and Outcomes

All participants in this study were followed every 4 weeks during the treatment, at the end of the therapy, and at week 12 posttreatment. During all visits, physical examination and biochemical evaluation were performed, and adherence to treatment and possible adverse events were analyzed. HCV RNA testing was performed at baseline, at 4 weeks, and at the end of the treatment (EOT). To assess the efficacy of the therapy, a sustained virological response (SVR12) was evaluated based on negative testing for HCV viral load using an RT-PCR method at week 12 posttreatment. Nonresponders were defined as patients with persistent HCV during treatment, and relapsers were considered as cases in which a reappearance of HCV RNA after its previous disappearance during or after the therapy occurred. Biochemical serum testing was performed using commercially available laboratory kits. For both alanine and aspartate aminotransferase (ALT and AST) serum levels, 40 IU/L was considered an upper limit of normal. Liver METAVIR fibrosis was assessed by the FibroScan device (Echosens, Paris, France) [16]. Transient elastography

(TE) examination was performed in all patients on the day the patient started treatment, and in patients presenting with significant fibrosis (F $\geq$ 2), it was also performed at week 12 posttreatment. Body mass index standard deviation (SD) scores (BMI z-scores) were calculated according to the WHO (Geneva, Switzerland) Child Growth Standards and Growth reference data using the WHO anthropometric calculator AnthroPlus v.1.0.4.

2.2. Statistical Analysis

Data distribution was evaluated with the Kolmogorov–Smirnov test before elaboration. Qualitative variables were reported as absolute and relative (percentage) frequencies. Quantitative variables were described as medians (interquartile ranges, IQRs), according to their non-parametric distribution. To compare continuous variables between more than two groups, repeated measures analysis of variance (ANOVA) testing was performed. A two-sided *p*-value of <0.05 was considered to indicate significance. All statistical analyses were performed using MedCalc Statistical Software version 20.009 (MedCalc, Ostend, Belgium).

2.3. Ethical Statement

The local ethics committee of the Medical University of Warsaw, Poland, approved this study (Number of approval: KB/87/2019; date of approval: 13 May 2019). Written informed consent was collected from all the patients and/or their parents/guardians before their inclusion in the study. The investigation was performed in accordance with the ethical standards in the 1964 Declaration of Helsinki and its later amendments.

3. Results

3.1. Study Group

Between August 2019 and December 2020, 37 patients qualified for treatment with LDV/SOF. Most of them were infected with genotype 1 HCV (26 with 1b; 4 with 1a; and 2 with undefined 1). Two patients were coinfected with human immunodeficiency virus (HIV) and had received effective antiretroviral treatment. One patient had evidence of previous hepatitis B virus infection (HBV): detectable anti-HBc antibodies with negative HBs antigen testing. Baseline liver stiffness measurement (LSM) revealed significant fibrosis (F $\geq$ 2 points in METAVIR scale) in 4/37 (11%) patients, including 3/37 (8%) with compensated cirrhosis (Child–Pugh class A). Two of these cirrhotic patients were infected with genotype 1b HCV, and they had a history of previous ineffective treatment with interferon and ribavirin. Thus, they were qualified for 24 weeks of LDV/SOF therapy. The baseline characteristics of the study group are presented in Table 1.

3.2. Efficacy of the Treatment

After four weeks of treatment, HCV RNA was undetectable in 31/37 (84%) patients and detectable in 6/37 (16%) patients, ranging between 14 and 942 IU/L (Figure 1). At the EOT, HCV RNA was undetectable in 31/37 (84%) patients, including 4 of the 6 patients with detectable HCV viral load after 4 weeks of therapy. In the remaining 6 cases, the evaluation was not performed due to the ongoing coronavirus disease 2019 (COVID-19) pandemic. Assessment of SVR12 was performed in 36/37 cases; however, in 21 participants, the evaluation of the SVR was postponed from 3 to 12 months as a result of the disruption caused by the COVID-19 pandemic. One patient (infected with genotype 1b, with cirrhosis) was lost to follow-up after week 4 of treatment when his HCV RNA was undetectable. However, home delivery of LDV/SOF was arranged for him, and he completed the 24-week therapy.

The overall intention-to-treat SVR12 rate in this group was 36/37 (97%). All the patients who completed the full protocol and were evaluated at least 12 weeks after the end of treatment achieved SVR12 (36/36, 100%) (Table 2). Intention-to-treat and per-protocol analyses of SVR12 according to the HCV genotype, baseline liver fibrosis, duration of the treatment, and previous ineffective treatment with interferon and ribavirin are presented in Table 2. There were no cases of treatment nonresponse or relapse in our study group.

Table 1. Baseline characteristics of 37 patients with chronic HCV infection treated with ledipasvir/sofosbuvir (LDV/SOF).

Characteristics		Number (%) or Median (IQR)
Sex	Male	23 (62)
	Female	14 (38)
Age	Median (IQR)	15 (12; 16)
HCV genotype	1	32 (86)
	4	5 (14)
Mode of infection	Mother-to-child transmission	30 (81)
	Unknown	7 (19)
Previous ineffective treatment with interferon plus ribavirin	Yes	14 (38)
	No	23 (62)
BMI	Median (IQR)	20.4 (17.7; 22.5)
BMI z-score	Median (IQR)	0.23 (−0.65; 0.83)
ALT	IU/mL, median (IQR)	37 (30; 48)
AST	IU/mL, median (IQR)	36 (32; 48)
HCV viral load	IU/mL, median (IQR)	5.83×10^5 (1.8×10^5; 12.6×10^5)
Liver fibrosis (LSM corresponding to METAVIR scale)	F0/F1	33 (89)
	F2	1 (3)
	F3	0
	F4	3 (8)
Anti-HIV	Positive	2 (5)
Anti-HBc total	Positive	1 (3)
Duration of LDV/SOF treatment	12 weeks	35 (95)
	24 weeks	2 (5)

ALT—alanine aminotransferase; AST—aspartate aminotransferase; LSM—liver stiffness measurement.

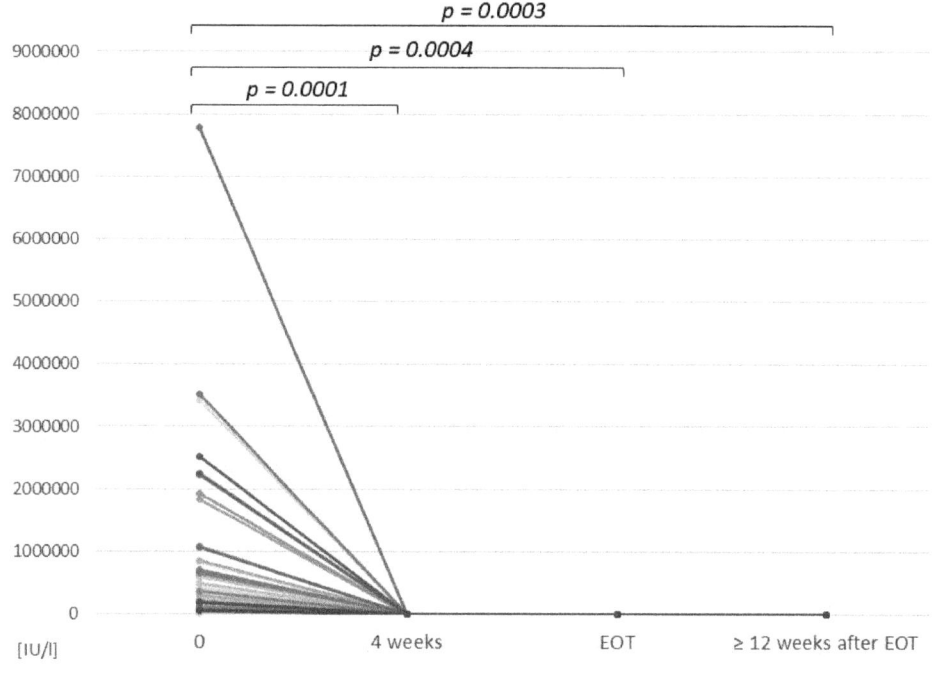

Figure 1. HCV viral load in 37 patients treated with LDV/SOF at baseline, at 4 weeks of treatment, at the end of treatment, and ≥ posttreatment week 12. EOT—end of treatment. Data at EOT were available for 31 patients.

Table 2. Efficacy of LDV/SOF treatment in 37 adolescents with CHC (intention-to-treat and per-protocol analysis).

Patient Characteristics		Number	SVR12 (ITT)	SVR12 (PP)
Overall		36/37	97%	100%
HCV genotype	1	31/32	97%	100%
	4	5/5	100%	100%
Baseline liver fibrosis (METAVIR)	F0/1	33/33	100%	100%
	F ≥ 2	3/4	75%	100%
Duration of LDV/SOF treatment	12 weeks	35/35	100%	100%
	24 weeks	1/2	50%	100%
Previous ineffective treatment with interferon and ribavirin	Yes	13/14	93%	100%
	No	23/23	100%	100%

ITT—intention-to-treat; PP—per-protocol analysis; SVR12—sustained virological response.

A significant decrease in both ALT and AST serum levels was observed in the subsequent weeks of the treatment and at SVR assessment compared to baseline (Figure 2A,B).

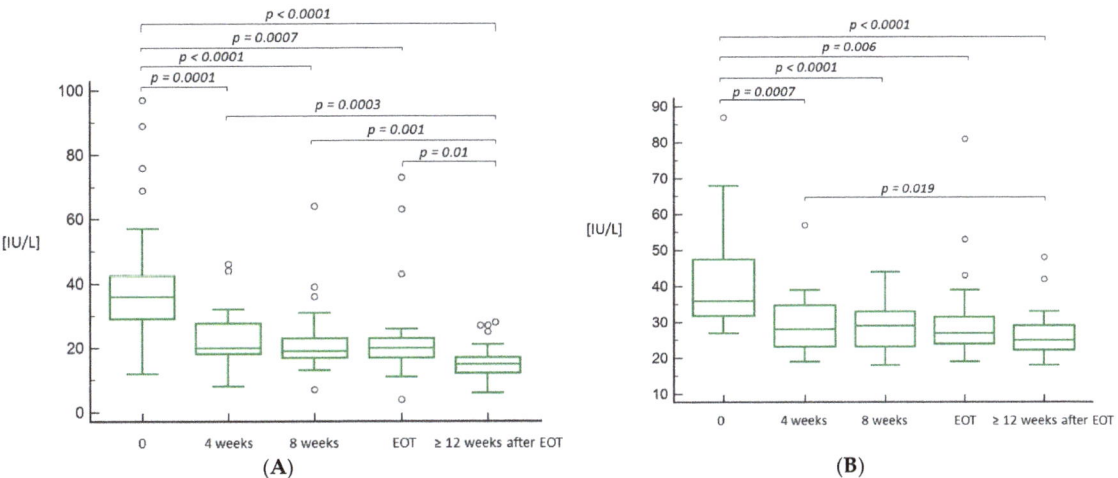

Figure 2. Box-and-whisker plots for alanine aminotransferase (**A**) and aspartate aminotransferase (**B**) levels during and after treatment with LDV/SOF. The top and bottom of each box are the 25th and 75th percentiles. The line through the box is the median, and the error bars are the maximum and minimum. (**A**) 0—start of treatment; EOT—end of treatment. (**B**) 0—start of treatment; EOT—end of treatment.

3.3. Tolerability and Safety of the Treatment

All 37 patients received treatment with the oral fixed-dose tablet of LDV/SOF (400/90 mg) once daily, and they all completed the treatment. No patient declared omission of any drug dose or delay in the admission of the drug dose longer than 3 h. The treatment was well tolerated. No serious adverse events were observed in this group. Overall, 11/37 (30%) patients complained of any adverse event, with fatigue as the most common (5/37, 14%). Other observed side effects of the treatment are listed in Table 3. Six patients (16%) suffered from upper respiratory tract infections during the treatment. In addition, two episodes of alcohol intoxication were reported in the study participants receiving treatment.

Table 3. Side effects of LDV/SOF treatment in 37 patients.

Symptom	Frequency, Number (%)
Any	11 (30)
Fatigue	5 (14)
Headache	4 (11)
Sleepiness	2 (5)
Diarrhea	2 (5)

4. Discussion

Our study revealed a 100% efficacy and a suitable safety profile of LDV/SOF treatment in children aged 12 to 17 years infected with genotypes 1 and 4 HCV. This therapy has been approved by the FDA and EMA for use in children aged 3 years and older with CHC based on the results of three open-label single-arm clinical trials [8–10]. However, one of the biggest problems of clinical trials is selection bias, which may lead to a mismatch between the trial population and real-world patients. Thus, their results should be confirmed by real-life studies, which would also include specific subgroups of patients, e.g., with liver cirrhosis, HIV/HCV, or HIV/HBV coinfections. In a recently published systematic review with meta-analysis on the efficacy and safety of different DAAs (including LDV/SOF) in children and adolescents with CHC, Indolfi et al. [13] demonstrated that among 39 included studies (both clinical trials and real-life studies) on 1796 subjects, the pooled SVR12 proportion among patients receiving all doses of the therapy was 100% (95% confidence interval 100–100). Among patients who received at least one dose of DAA, the lowest efficacy of the treatment (83%) was reported for children with cirrhosis [13]. However, it should be emphasized that the number of performed studies on LDV/SOF treatment in children and adolescents remains limited, and there is a need for further research in this area. We identified 15 papers (both clinical trials and real-life studies) that analyzed SVR in almost 1000 pediatric patients treated with LDV/SOF (Table 4). In all of these investigations, the treatment was effective in at least 95% of patients, which is consistent with our results, showing SVR in 97% of participants. The few patients who did not achieve SVR were (as in our study) lost to follow-up. There were only single cases described of relapse after the treatment [9]. Pooled data from the 15 abovementioned studies and our investigation on 1016 patients revealed an SVR rate of 98.6% for all genotypes, including 98.4% for patients infected with genotype 1, 75% for genotype 3, and 98.9% for genotype 4 HCV (Table 4). Lower SVR rates for genotype 3 may result from a small number of patients in this group (only 4). It is worth emphasizing that real-life studies on LDV/SOF treatment in children were mainly performed in Egypt; thus, they mainly investigated patients infected with genotype 4 HCV [17–23]. Studies analyzing the efficacy of LDV/SOF in children infected with genotype 1 are less represented. In a recently published Italian study by Serranti et al. [24], 78 patients were included: 64 infected with genotype 1; 2 with genotype 3; and 12 with genotype 4 HCV. The overall intention-to-treat SVR12 rate was 97.4%, but per-protocol analysis revealed SVR12 rates of 100% overall and separately for all genotypes (1, 3, and 4 HCV). This observation was similar to our results: our per-protocol SVR12 rates were 100% irrespective of the HCV genotype, duration of the treatment, previous treatment experience, or baseline extent of liver fibrosis (Table 2). It is worth emphasizing that the treatment was effective in cirrhotic patients and in two participants coinfected with HIV, as described in detail in another paper [25]. In addition, one of our patients had evidence of past HBV infection with detectable anti-HBc total antibodies. He was closely monitored during and after the treatment, and reactivation of the HBV infection did not occur (ALT and AST levels were normal, HBV DNA was undetectable during and after the treatment) [26]. In a large cohort of adults with HCV/HBV coinfection treated with DAAs, the risk of HBV reactivation in HBsAg-negative/anti-HBc-positive patients was only 0.16% [26]. To avoid HBV reactivation in patients with serologic evidence of a previous or current HBV infection, the clinical and laboratory signs of a hepatitis flare or HBV reactivation should be monitored during treatment with DAAs and posttreatment follow-up. Despite the fact that elevation of the ALT and AST serum levels in patients with CHC is not obligatory and usually not persistent, we found a significant decrease in their levels during the course and after the treatment, which is consistent with observations of the Italian cohort [24].

Table 4. Summary of the studies on LDV/SOF efficacy in pediatric patients with chronic hepatitis C.

No	Patients Age Range (Years)	Number of Participants	HCV Genotype	Duration of Treatment (Weeks)	Number of Patients Achieving SVR12 (%)	Reference
1	12–18	40	4	12	100	El-Karaksy et al. 2018 [19]
2	12–18	46	NA	12	98	Fouad et al. 2020 [27]
3	12–17	100	1	12	98	Balistreri et al. 2017 [8]
4	12–17	144	4	12	99	El-Khayat et al. 2018 [21]
5	12–17	14	1	8	100	Serranti et al. 2019 [28]
6	12–17	78	1, 3, 4	8, 12 or 24	97.4	Serranti et al. 2021 [24]
7	12–17	157	4	8 or 12	98	El-Khayat et al. 2019 [20]
8	12–17	65	4	12	100	Makhlouf et al. 2021 [29]
9	11–17	51	4	12	100	Fouad et al. 2019 [30]
10	9–12	100	4	12	100	El-Araby et al. 2019 [18]
11	6–12	20	4	12	95	El-Shabrawi et al. 2018 [22]
12	6–11	92	1, 3, 4	12 or 24	99	Murray et al. 2018 [9]
13	4–10	30	4	8	100	Behairy et al. 2020 [17]
14	3–6	22	4	8 or 12	100	Kamal et al. 2020 [23]
15	3–5	34	1, 4	12	97	Schwarz et al. 2020 [10]
Overall and According to the HCV Genotype						
16	3–18	1016	1, 3, 4	8, 12 or 24	98.6	*
17	3–17	317	1	8, 12 or 24	98.4	**
18	6–17	4	3	24	75	***
19	3–18	649	4	8 or 12	98.9	****

* cumulative data from studies No. 1–4 and 6–15 and from our study (participants of study No. 5 are included in study No. 6); ** cumulative data from the above studies No. 3, 6, 12, 15 and from our study; *** cumulative data from the above studies No. 6 and 12; **** cumulative data from the above studies No. 1, 4, 6–15 and from our study, SVR—sustained virological response.

The treatment with LDV/SOF was well tolerated. No participant discontinued the treatment due to side effects. However, a number of patients complained of the large size of the tablets, which were difficult to swallow. No patient complained of the taste of the drug, which was reported in the cohort of younger children (receiving pellets) [10]. According to the results of the meta-analysis performed by Indolfi et al. the most common adverse events reported in children and adolescents receiving DAAs include headache (19.9%), fatigue/asthenia (13.9%), nausea (8.1%), abdominal pain (7.0%), diarrhea (4.8%), cough (4.0%), and vomiting (2.6%) [13]. Similar side effects were observed in our cohort, with fatigue as the most common (14%). No serious adverse events were reported in the meta-analysis or in our study [13].

Teenagers constitute a special group of pediatric patients; they usually have a sense of immortality, they want to be independent, and their adherence to longer-lasting therapies and obligatory checkups is usually poor. Thus, the value of the study is the fact that it was possible to carry out the entire therapy program and follow-up in 36/37 patients. This indicates that treatment based on DAAs is short and well tolerated by this specific age group of patients.

The treatment duration in our study was established according to the ESPGHAN guidelines, with a minimum duration of 12 weeks [15]. However, there is some evidence based on four reported studies (Table 4) that shortening the duration of LDV/SOF treatment to 8 weeks is equally effective [17,20,24,27]. In the studies by Serranti et al. [24,28], 17 patients in total who were infected with genotype 1 HCV, treatment-naïve, noncirrhotic, and with baseline HCV viral load below 6,000,000 IU/mL were treated with LDF/SOF for 8 weeks. The SVR12 rate in this group was 17/17 (100%). Our data showing that most of the patients had undetectable HCV RNA at 4 weeks of treatment may, to some extent, support shortening LDF/SOF treatment in adolescents.

Our study has some limitations. First, the number of included patients was relatively low. Our study group represents no more than 10% of all pediatric HCV cases diagnosed in Poland during the last decade (2). However, all consecutive patients infected with genotypes 1 and 4 HCV referring to our department were included. To the best of our knowledge, this is the second report on a real-life experience with LDV/SOF in adolescents from Europe, demonstrating the efficacy in participants infected with genotype 1 HCV. As presented in Table 4, studies on the large groups of pediatric patients in this area are unavailable. In addition, our 32 patients infected with genotype 1 HCV represented 10% of all of the pediatric study participants with genotype 1 treated with LDV/SOF (Table 4). Second, gaps in the available data resulting from the disruption caused by the COVID-19 pandemic should be mentioned. However, treatment was completed by all of the patients despite the pandemic, which was achieved thanks to the several efforts that were made to prioritize patient care in our children with CHC, following our own guidelines in this field [31]. In addition, DAA therapies are relatively simple, short, and safe. Thus, less frequent monitoring of patients receiving them might be considered.

In conclusion, the results of this real-life study confirm previous observations based mainly on clinical trials of a suitable efficacy and safety profile of LDV/SOF for the treatment of CHC genotypes 1 and 4 in adolescents, regardless of baseline liver fibrosis or previous ineffective antiviral treatment experience.

Author Contributions: Conceptualization, M.P.-Ś.; methodology, M.P.-Ś.; formal analysis, M.P.-Ś.; investigation, M.P.-Ś., A.D., and M.A.; data curation, M.P.-Ś., A.D. and M.A.; writing—original draft preparation, M.P.-Ś.; writing—review and editing, M.P.-Ś.; visualization, M.P.-Ś.; supervision, M.M. All authors have read and agreed to the published version of the manuscript.

Funding: This research received no external funding. The therapeutic program was available courtesy of the donation of LDV/SOF by the pharmaceutical company (Gilead Sciences Poland Sp. Z o. o., Warsaw, Poland). The pharmaceutical company did not have any role in performing the study, nor in writing or approving this manuscript.

Institutional Review Board Statement: The investigation was performed in accordance with the ethical standards in the 1964 Declaration of Helsinki and its later amendments. The local ethics committee of the Medical University of Warsaw approved this study (No KB/87/2019; date of approval: 13 May 2019).

Informed Consent Statement: Written informed consent was collected from all the patients and/or their parents/guardians before their inclusion in the study.

Data Availability Statement: The datasets used and analyzed during the current study are available from the corresponding author upon reasonable request.

Acknowledgments: The authors would like to thank the following clinicians for referring their patients for participation in the POLAC Project: Anna Gorczyca, Maria Rokitka, Ewelina Gowin, Joanna Łasecka-Zadrożna, Józef Rudnicki, Mariola Purzyńska, Agnieszka Ogrodnik, Anna Mania, Magdalena Figlerowicz, Barbara Hasiec, Agnieszka Krasiukianis, and Ewa Majda-Stanisławska.

Conflicts of Interest: The authors declare no conflict of interest.

References

1. Schmelzer, J.; Dugan, E.; Blach, S.; Coleman, S.B.; Cai, Z.; DePaola, M.; Estes, C.; Gamkrelidze, I.; Jerabek, K.; Ma, S.; et al. Global prevalence of hepatitis C virus in children in 2018: A modelling study. *Lancet Gastroenterol. Hepatol.* **2020**, *5*, 374–392. [CrossRef]
2. National Institute of Public Health. Reports on Cases of Infectious Diseases and Poisonings in Poland. Available online: http://wwwold.pzh.gov.pl/oldpage/epimeld/index_a.html#01 (accessed on 27 July 2021).
3. Modin, L.; Arshad, A.; Wilkes, B.; Benselin, J.; Lloyd, C.; Irving, W.L.; Kelly, D.A. Epidemiology and natural history of hepatitis C virus infection among children and young people. *J. Hepatol.* **2019**, *70*, 371–378. [CrossRef] [PubMed]
4. Pokorska-Śpiewak, M.; Dobrzeniecka, A.; Lipińska, M.; Tomasik, A.; Aniszewska, M.; Marczyńska, M. Liver Fibrosis Evaluated With Transient Elastography in 35 Children With Chronic Hepatitis C Virus Infection. *Pediatr. Infect. Dis. J.* **2021**, *40*, 103–108. [CrossRef]

5. Turkova, A.; Volynets, G.V.; Crichton, S.; Skvortsova, T.A.; Panfilova, V.N.; Rogozina, N.V.; Khavkin, A.I.; Tumanova, E.L.; Indolfi, G.; Thorne, C. Advanced liver disease in Russian children and adolescents with chronic hepatitis C. *J. Viral Hepat.* **2019**, *26*, 881–892. [CrossRef]
6. Younossi, Z.M.; Stepanova, M.; Schwarz, K.B.; Wirth, S.; Rosenthal, P.; Gonzalez-Peralta, R.; Murray, K.; Henry, L.; Hunt, S. Quality of life in adolescents with hepatitis C treated with sofosbuvir and ribavirin. *J. Viral Hepat.* **2017**, *25*, 354–362. [CrossRef]
7. United Nations. Transforming Our World: The 2030 Agenda for Sustainable Development. New York, United Nations. 2015. Available online: https://sdgs.un.org/2030agenda (accessed on 27 July 2021).
8. Balistreri, W.F.; Murray, K.F.; Rosenthal, P.; Bansal, S.; Lin, C.H.; Kersey, K.; Massetto, B.; Zhu, Y.; Kanwar, B.; German, P.; et al. The safety and effectiveness of ledipasvir-sofosbuvir in adolescents 12–17 years old with hepatitis C virus genotype 1 infection. *Hepatology* **2017**, *66*, 371–378. [CrossRef] [PubMed]
9. Murray, K.F.; Balistreri, W.F.; Bansal, S.; Whitworth, S.; Evans, H.M.; Gonzalez-Peralta, R.P.; Wen, J.; Massetto, B.; Kersey, K.; Shao, J.; et al. Safety and Efficacy of Ledipasvir-Sofosbuvir With or Without Ribavirin for Chronic Hepatitis C in Children Ages 6–11. *Hepatology* **2018**, *68*, 2158–2166. [CrossRef] [PubMed]
10. Schwarz, K.B.; Rosenthal, P.; Murray, K.F.; Honegger, J.R.; Hardikar, W.; Hague, R.; Mittal, N.; Massetto, B.; Brainard, D.M.; Hsueh, C.; et al. Ledipasvir-Sofosbuvir for 12 Weeks in Children 3 to <6 Years Old With Chronic Hepatitis C. *Hepatology* **2019**, *71*, 422–430. [CrossRef]
11. El-Sayed, M.H.; Indolfi, G. Hepatitis C Virus Treatment in Children: A Challenge for Hepatitis C Virus Elimination. *Semin. Liver Dis.* **2020**, *40*, 213–224. [CrossRef] [PubMed]
12. Indolfi, G.; Easterbrook, P.; Dusheiko, G.; El-Sayed, M.H.; Jonas, M.M.; Thorne, C.; Bulterys, M.; Siberry, G.; Walsh, N.; Chang, M.-H.; et al. Hepatitis C virus infection in children and adolescents. *Lancet Gastroenterol. Hepatol.* **2019**, *4*, 477–487. [CrossRef]
13. Indolfi, G.; Giometto, S.; Serranti, D.; Bettiol, A.; Bigagli, E.; De Masi, S.; Lucenteforte, E. Systematic review with meta-analysis: The efficacy and safety of direct-acting antivirals in children and adolescents with chronic hepatitis C virus infection. *Aliment. Pharmacol. Ther.* **2020**, *52*, 1125–1133. [PubMed]
14. Rogers, M.E.; Balistreri, W.F. Cascade of care for children and adolescents with chronic hepatitis C. *World J. Gastroenterol.* **2021**, *27*, 1117–1131. [CrossRef]
15. Indolfi, G.; Hierro, L.; Dezsofi, A.; Jahnel, J.; Debray, D.; Hadzic, N.; Czubowski, P.; Gupte, G.; Mozer-Glassberg, Y.; Van Der Woerd, W.; et al. Treatment of Chronic Hepatitis C Virus Infection in Children: A Position Paper by the Hepatology Committee of European Society of Paediatric Gastroenterology, Hepatology and Nutrition. *J. Pediatr. Gastroenterol. Nutr.* **2018**, *66*, 505–515. [CrossRef] [PubMed]
16. Castéra, L.; Vergniol, J.; Foucher, J.; Le Bail, B.; Chanteloup, E.; Haaser, M.; Darriet, M.; Couzigou, P.; de Lédinghen, V. Prospective comparison of transient elastography, Fibrotest, APRI, and liver biopsy for the assessment of fibrosis in chronic hepatitis C. *Gastroenterology* **2005**, *128*, 343–350. [CrossRef] [PubMed]
17. Behairy, B.E.; El-Araby, H.A.; El-Guindi, M.A.; Basiouny, H.M.; Fouad, O.A.; Ayoub, B.A.; Marei, A.M.; Sira, M.M. Safety and Efficacy of 8 Weeks Ledipasvir/Sofosbuvir for Chronic Hepatitis C Genotype 4 in Children Aged 4–10 Years. *J. Pediatr.* **2020**, *219*, 106–110. [CrossRef] [PubMed]
18. El-Araby, H.A.; Behairy, B.E.; El-Guindi, M.A.; Adawy, N.M.; Allam, A.A.; Sira, A.M.; Khedr, M.A.; Elhenawy, I.A.; Sobhy, G.A.; Basiouny, H.E.D.M.; et al. Generic sofosbuvir/ledipasvir for the treatment of genotype 4 chronic hepatitis C in Egyptian children (9–12 years) and adolescents. *Hepatol. Int.* **2019**, *13*, 706–714. [CrossRef]
19. El-Karaksy, H.; Mogahed, E.A.; Abdullatif, H.; Ghobrial, C.; El-Raziky, M.S.; El-Koofy, N.; El-Shabrawi, M.; Ghita, H.; Baroudy, S.; Okasha, S. Sustained Viral Response in Genotype 4 Chronic Hepatitis C Virus-infected Children and Adolescents Treated With Sofosbuvir/Ledipasvir. *J. Pediatr. Gastroenterol. Nutr.* **2018**, *67*, 626–630. [CrossRef]
20. El-Khayat, H.; Kamal, E.M.; Yakoot, M.; Gawad, M.A.; Kamal, N.; El Shabrawi, M.; El-Shabrawi, M.; Ghita, H.; Baroudy, S.; Okasha, S. Effectiveness of 8-week sofosbuvir/ledipasvir in the adolescent chronic hepatitis C-infected patients. *Eur. J. Gastroenterol. Hepatol.* **2019**, *31*, 1004–1009. [CrossRef]
21. El-Khayat, H.; Kamal, E.M.; El-Sayed, M.H.; El-Shabrawi, M.; Ayoub, H.; Rizk, A.; Maher, M.; El Sheemy, R.Y.; Fouad, Y.M.; Attia, D. The effectiveness and safety of ledipasvir plus sofosbuvir in adolescents with chronic hepatitis C virus genotype 4 infection: A real-world experience. *Aliment. Pharmacol. Ther.* **2018**, *47*, 838–844. [CrossRef]
22. El-Shabrawi, M.; Kamal, N.M.; El-Khayat, H.R.; Kamal, E.M.; AbdelGawad, M.M.A.H.; Yakoot, M. A pilot single arm observational study of sofosbuvir/ledipasvir (200 + 45 mg) in 6- to 12- year old children. *Aliment. Pharmacol. Ther.* **2018**, *47*, 1699–1704. [CrossRef]
23. Kamal, E.M.; El-Shabrawi, M.; El-Khayat, H.; Yakoot, M.; Sameh, Y.; Fouad, Y.; Attia, D. Effects of sofosbuvir/ledipasvir therapy on chronic hepatitis C virus genotype 4, infected children of 3-6 years of age. *Liver Int.* **2019**, *40*, 319–323. [CrossRef]
24. Serranti, D.; Nebbia, G.; Cananzi, M.; Nicastro, E.; Di Dato, F.; Nuti, F.; Garazzino, S.; Silvestro, E.; Giacomet, V.; Forlanini, F.; et al. Efficacy of Sofosbuvir/Ledipasvir in Adolescents With Chronic Hepatitis C Genotypes 1, 3, and 4: A Real-world Study. *J. Pediatr. Gastroenterol. Nutr.* **2020**, *72*, 95–100. [CrossRef] [PubMed]
25. Pokorska-Śpiewak, M.; Dobrzeniecka, A.; Ołdakowska, A.; Marczyńska, M. Effective Treatment of Chronic Hepatitis C Virus Infection with Ledipasvir/Sofosbuvir in 2 Teenagers with HIV Coinfection: A Brief Report. *Pediatr. Infect. Dis. J.* **2021**. [CrossRef]
26. Jaroszewicz, J.; Pawłowska, M.; Simon, K.; Zarębska-Michaluk, D.; Lorenc, B.; Klapaczyński, J.; Tudrujek-Zdunek, M.; Sitko, M.; Mazur, W.; Janczewska, E.; et al. Low risk of HBV reactivation in a large European cohort of HCV/HBV coinfected patients treated with DAA. *Expert Rev. Anti-Infective Ther.* **2020**, *18*, 1045–1054. [CrossRef]

27. Fouad, H.M.; Sabry, M.A.; Ahmed, A.; Hassany, M.; Al Soda, M.F.; Aziz, H.A. Generic Ledipasvir-Sofosbuvir Treatment for Adolescents With Chronic Hepatitis C Virus Infection. *J. Pediatr. Infect. Dis. Soc.* **2019**, *9*, 386–389. [CrossRef] [PubMed]
28. Serranti, D.; Dodi, I.; Nicastro, E.; Cangelosi, A.M.; Riva, S.; Ricci, S.; Bartolini, E.; Trapani, S.; Mastrangelo, G.; Vajro, P.; et al. Shortened 8-Week Course of Sofosbuvir/Ledipasvir Therapy in Adolescents With Chronic Hepatitis C Infection. *J. Pediatr. Gastroenterol. Nutr.* **2019**, *69*, 595–598. [CrossRef] [PubMed]
29. Makhlouf, N.A.; Abdelmalek, M.O.; Ibrahim, M.E.; Abu-Faddan, N.H.; Kheila, A.E.; Mahmoud, A.A. Ledipasvir/Sofosbuvir in Adolescents With Chronic Hepatitis C Genotype 4 With and Without Hematological Disorders: Virological Efficacy and Impact on Liver Stiffness. *J. Pediatric. Infect. Dis. Soc.* **2021**, *10*, 7–13. [CrossRef]
30. Fouad, H.M.; Ahmed Mohamed, A.; Sabry, M.; Abdel Aziz, H.; Eysa, B.; Rabea, M. The Effectiveness of Ledipasvir/Sofosbuvir in Youth With Genotype 4 Hepatitis C Virus: A Single Egyptian Center Study. *Pediatr Infect. Dis. J.* **2019**, *38*, 22–25. [CrossRef] [PubMed]
31. Pokorska-Śpiewak, M.; Śpiewak, M. Management of hepatitis C in children and adolescents during COVID-19 pandemic. *World J. Hepatol.* **2020**, *12*, 485–492. [CrossRef] [PubMed]

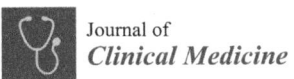

Article

The Netherlands Is on Track to Meet the World Health Organization Hepatitis C Elimination Targets by 2030

Marleen van Dijk [1,*], Sylvia M. Brakenhoff [2,†], Cas J. Isfordink [3,4,†], Wei-Han Cheng [5], Hans Blokzijl [6], Greet Boland [7], Anthonius S. M. Dofferhoff [8], Bart van Hoek [9], Cees van Nieuwkoop [10], Milan J. Sonneveld [2], Marc van der Valk [4], Joost P. H. Drenth [1] and Robert J. de Knegt [2]

[1] Department of Gastroenterology and Hepatology, Radboud University Medical Centre, 6525 GA Nijmegen, The Netherlands; joostphdrenth@cs.com
[2] Department of Gastroenterology and Hepatology, Erasmus University Medical Centre, 3015 GD Rotterdam, The Netherlands; s.brakenhoff@erasmusmc.nl (S.M.B.); m.j.sonneveld@erasmusmc.nl (M.J.S.); r.deknegt@erasmusmc.nl (R.J.d.K.)
[3] Department of Gastroenterology and Hepatology, University Medical Centre Utrecht, 3584 CX Utrecht, The Netherlands; c.j.isfordink-3@umcutrecht.nl
[4] Division of Infectious Diseases, Department of Internal Medicine, Amsterdam Infection & Immunity Institute, Amsterdam UMC, University of Amsterdam, 1105 AZ Amsterdam, The Netherlands; m.vandervalk@amsterdamumc.nl
[5] Health Economics and Outcomes Research, AbbVie Inc., North Chicago, IL 60064, USA; wei-han.cheng@abbvie.com
[6] Department of Gastroenterology and Hepatology, University Medical Centre Groningen, 9713 GZ Groningen, The Netherlands; h.blokzijl@umcg.nl
[7] Department of Medical Microbiology, University Medical Centre Utrecht, 3584 CX Utrecht, The Netherlands; g.j.boland@umcutrecht.nl
[8] Department of Internal Medicine, Canisius Wilhelmina Hospital, Radboud University Medical Centre, 6532 SZ Nijmegen, The Netherlands; a.dofferhoff@cwz.nl
[9] Department of Gastroenterology and Hepatology, Leiden University Medical Centre, 2333 ZA Leiden, The Netherlands; b.van_hoek@lumc.nl
[10] Department of Internal Medicine, Haga Teaching Hospital, 2545 AA The Hague, The Netherlands; c.vannieuwkoop@hagaziekenhuis.nl
* Correspondence: marleen.vandijk@radboudumc.nl
† These authors contributed equally.

Abstract: Background: The Netherlands strives for hepatitis C virus (HCV) elimination, in accordance with the World Health Organization targets. An accurate estimate when HCV elimination will be reached is elusive. We have embarked on a nationwide HCV elimination project (CELINE) that allowed us to harvest detailed data on the Dutch HCV epidemic. This study aims to provide a well-supported timeline towards HCV elimination in The Netherlands. Methods: A previously published Markov model was used, adopting published data and unpublished CELINE project data. Two main scenarios were devised. In the Status Quo scenario, 2020 diagnosis and treatment levels remained constant in subsequent years. In the Gradual Decline scenario, an annual decrease of 10% in both diagnoses and treatments was implemented, starting in 2020. WHO incidence target was disregarded, due to low HCV incidence in The Netherlands (≤5 per 100,000). Results: Following the Status Quo and Gradual Decline scenarios, The Netherlands would meet WHO's elimination targets by 2027 and 2032, respectively. From 2015 to 2030, liver-related mortality would be reduced by 97% in the Status Quo and 93% in the Gradual Decline scenario. Compared to the Status Quo scenario, the Gradual Decline scenario would result in 12 excess cases of decompensated cirrhosis, 18 excess cases of hepatocellular carcinoma, and 20 excess cases of liver-related death from 2020–2030. Conclusions: The Netherlands is on track to reach HCV elimination by 2030. However, it is vital that HCV elimination remains high on the agenda to ensure adequate numbers of patients are being diagnosed and treated.

Keywords: hepatitis C; HCV; elimination; model; COVID-19

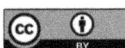

1. Introduction

Chronic viral hepatitis, if left untreated, leads to considerable morbidity and liver-related mortality [1]. Therefore, the World Health Organization (WHO) set ambitious hepatitis B (HBV) and C virus (HCV) elimination targets in 2016. The goal is to eliminate viral hepatitis as a public health threat by 2030, which is defined by the following targets: (1) 80% reduction in incidence, (2) 65% reduction in hepatitis-related mortality, (3) 90% diagnosis coverage, and (4) 80% treatment coverage [2]. The year 2015 serves as baseline for these targets. Many countries aim to reach these goals in time and elaborate efforts have been made to monitor progress towards elimination, often using mathematical models [3,4].

With regard to hepatitis C, it appears that only few countries are on track to meeting the WHO targets in time [5]. A recent modelling study, using the latest data on chronic HCV prevalence, and annual diagnosis and treatment levels in 45 high-income countries, suggests that only Australia, Canada, France, Germany, Iceland, Italy, Japan, Spain, Sweden, Switzerland, and the United Kingdom are currently on track [5]. Tailored HCV-specific national strategies, regional or national guidelines, national expert advisory groups and/or decentralized HCV screening likely keep these countries on a trajectory towards elimination.

The situation is different in The Netherlands. While there is a national plan that is endorsed by the Ministry of Health, the government has not allocated funds to aid its execution, and the plan itself lacks specific targets and accompanying interventions. Furthermore, The Netherlands does not yet have a nationwide hepatitis registry, complicating the ability to track our progress. However, physicians took the initiative to establish a national collaboration group (HepNed) to create the necessary infrastructure to eliminate HCV. HepNed has initiated several HCV elimination projects, such as CELINE and CAC.

CELINE, which stands for hepatitis C elimination in The Netherlands, is a nationwide retrieval project aiming to re-engage lost to follow-up HCV patients with care [6]. The project uses laboratory and patient records dating back 15 years from virtually all hepatitis treatment centers in The Netherlands. CAC, which stands for hepatitis C Chain of Addiction Care, is a project that aims to decentralize HCV care for people visiting addiction care services, one of the few remaining risk groups for chronic HCV infection in The Netherlands, even though transmission is very low [7]. Patients in several facilities all over The Netherlands are screened and linked to care, and data is collected throughout this process. These projects have provided us with high quality data on the current epidemiology of HCV in The Netherlands.

A recent study estimated that The Netherlands will reach the WHO HCV elimination targets by 2035 [5]. However, this study did not have access to the detailed epidemiologic data yielded from recent elimination projects. A previous Dutch modelling study from the pre-DAA era investigated various strategies to reduce the future HCV disease burden [8]. Many changes from their most effective strategy have since been implemented, including unrestricted access to direct-acting antivirals (DAA). Furthermore, various efforts to achieve viral hepatitis elimination have since been initiated. The aim of the present modelling study is therefore to evaluate the current timeline towards HCV elimination in The Netherlands.

2. Methods

2.1. The Model

We utilized a mathematical model developed by the Centre for Disease Analysis [4] to model the current progress towards HCV elimination as well as the effect of various interventions on HCV-associated outcomes. This model has been used extensively in various healthcare situations and countries [9–14]. Briefly, the Excel-based Markov model forecasts the future HCV-infected population and associated liver-related morbidity (decompensated cirrhosis and hepatocellular carcinoma) and mortality. The model uses an age- and gender-specific disease progression framework, previously detailed elsewhere [9]. It incorporates the WHO targets and forecasts when the country will reach these goals.

Ethical approval from an institutional review board was not required for the execution of this study.

2.2. Model Base-Case Input

The model requires various parameters as base-case input (Table 1). These input parameters were based on the literature and/or consensus from expert meetings with HCV physicians and public health (modelling) experts from the National Institute for Public Health and the Environment and from Municipal Health Services, and are described in Table 1 and in detail below.

Table 1. Base Case Model Inputs.

Variable	Input	Source
Size of overall population (2016)	16,890,864	United Nations [15]
Ever-infected patients with chronic HCV (up to 2016)	23,647	2016 prevalence [16], adjusted to include people < 15 years old
Total number of viraemic patients (2016)	11,057	Based on the adjusted 2016 prevalence [16] and the estimated number of cured patients up to 2016
Ever-diagnosed patients (up to 2016)	16,533	CELINE data (unpublished)
Total number of diagnosed patients (2016)	3963	Based on CELINE data and the estimated number of cured patients up to 2016
Number of annual newly diagnosed patients (2016)	700	CELINE data (unpublished)
Number of annual treated patients 2016 2017 2018 2019	 2647 1173 988 776	GIP database [17]
Fibrosis stage restriction (2016)	$\geq$F0	No treatment restrictions since 2016
Maximum age eligible for treatment (2016)	85+	No treatment restrictions since 2016
Average SVR (2016)	95%	See Supplementary File S1

2.2.1. Viraemic Prevalence

The prevalence of chronic HCV infection in The Netherlands in 2016 [16] was estimated by using the workbook method, originally developed to estimate the HIV/AIDS prevalence in low endemic countries with concentrated epidemics [18]. This study estimates that 22,885 people aged 15 years and older were ever chronically infected with HCV [16]. We adjusted this prevalence to include people aged 14 years or younger (Table 1), based on the age distribution detailed elsewhere [8].

The number of viraemic individuals in 2016 was calculated by subtracting the number of patients cured up to 2016 from the adjusted 2016 prevalence estimate. Treatment data were obtained from the GIP database, a web-based database from the Dutch National Health Care Institute that contains data on physician-prescribed medication in outpatient care [17]. Supplementary Table S1 displays (pegylated) interferon and DAA prescriptions from 2000–2016. These data reflect the annual total number of individual users, independent of treatment indication. As indications for (pegylated) interferon-based therapy expand beyond chronic HCV, we revised this data to reflect the treated and cured HCV population (Supplementary File S1 and Table S2). This resulted in an estimated population of 12,590 cured patients, leading to a baseline of 11,057 viraemic patients in 2016 (Table 1).

2.2.2. HCV Incidence

The biggest influx of new HCV infections in The Netherlands is generated by first-generation migrants from HCV-endemic countries. An estimated 400 new chronic infections are introduced to The Netherlands yearly due to migration, based on annual migration statistics and published prevalence data [19,20]. The model incorporates these infections into the HCV incidence. True HCV incidence, due to active transmission, is estimated to be very low in The Netherlands. People who inject(ed) drugs (PWID) used to be a major HCV risk group in The Netherlands. However, due to the implementation of several successful harm reduction strategies, accompanied by a change in drug use culture, HCV incidence has declined [21]. After 2000, the primary risk group for HCV infection was no longer PWID, but men who have sex with men (MSM) [22,23]. Nowadays, almost all acute HCV cases occur among MSM [7]. The National Institute for Public Health and the Environment data from the previous 10 years show that, on average, the annual number of acute HCV cases is 54 (range 30–67) [7]. The incidence of HCV re-infection has increased over the last few years, with 26 re-infections reported in 2019 as compared to 2 in 2016 [24]. A recent study suggests that the WHO HCV incidence target may be hard to reach in countries where HCV incidence is already low [25]. The authors propose an adapted incidence goal: annual incidence ≤ 5 per 100,000 people. This adapted incidence goal has already been met, both in 2016 and 2019 [7,24]. We have therefore disregarded the WHO incidence goal incorporated in the model.

2.2.3. Number of Diagnosed Individuals

Numbers of ever-diagnosed and annually diagnosed patients were based on CELINE project data (unpublished) [6]. Approximately 70% of ever-infected patients received a formal diagnosis, resulting in 3963 diagnosed but untreated people remaining at large in 2016 (Table 1). During 2016–2019, an average of 728 patients were newly diagnosed with viraemic HCV annually. This number corresponds with the number of 700 used in a similar modelling study by Hatzakis et al. [26].

2.2.4. Number of Treated Individuals

Treatment data were obtained from the GIP database [17]. Data on HCV therapy and cure from 2000–2015 are presented in Supplementary File S1. Prior to 2016, DAA treatment was reserved for people with advanced disease (patients with F3 fibrosis or cirrhosis, liver transplant patients or candidates, and patients with severe extrahepatic manifestations). Since November 2015, all official restrictions on DAA treatment were lifted, resulting in widely available and reimbursed HCV treatment for everyone with health insurance. Therefore, SVR was assumed to be >95% during and after 2016. A total of 776 people were treated with DAAs in 2019 (see Supplementary Tables S2 and S3).

2.3. Model Scenarios

Our aim was to evaluate the Dutch timeline towards HCV elimination, starting in 2020. First, we intended to develop a scenario maintaining our elimination efforts on the same level as in 2019 ("Status Quo" scenario). As this might be an optimistic scenario, we also wanted to incorporate a scenario in which a yearly reduction in elimination efforts was implemented ("Gradual Decline" scenario). We also performed a sensitivity analysis, implementing a larger reduction in elimination efforts.

During the execution of this study, Coronavirus Disease 2019 (COVID-19) emerged, leading to a serious strain on healthcare in our country with devastating effects on non-COVID care [27,28]. Therefore, we implemented a substantial decrease in elimination efforts in both scenarios. This decrease was implemented for two years, as a one-year delay was deemed too optimistic. This two-year delay in the Status Quo scenario resulted in the Two-year COVID-19 Delay scenario, whereas the delay in the Gradual Decline scenario resulted in the Post-recovery Gradual Decline Scenario. All scenarios are detailed below.

2.3.1. Status Quo Scenario

The annual number of treated patients peaked in 2015, just after the introduction of DAAs, but declined continuously thereafter (Supplementary Figure S1). For the Status

Quo scenario, we assumed that this decline would reach its plateau in 2020. We therefore reduced the number of annual treatments with 10% as compared to 2019, and applied a similar reduction to the annual number of diagnosed patients. From 2021 onwards, these numbers were modelled to remain equal to 2020. The scenario inputs can be found in Supplementary Table S4.

2.3.2. Gradual Decline Scenario

In the second scenario ("Gradual Decline"), we assumed a continuous reduction of 10% per year in both the number of annual newly diagnosed and treated patients, starting in 2021. The Gradual Decline scenario model inputs can be found in Supplementary Table S5. Furthermore, a sensitivity analysis was run on this scenario, to assess the impact of a larger reduction in elimination efforts ("Sensitivity Analysis"). An annual reduction of 15% in newly diagnosed and treated patients was therefore implemented, starting in 2021. Other scenario variables were not altered. The Sensitivity Analysis model inputs can be found in Supplementary Table S6.

2.3.3. COVID-19 Scenarios

A recent study from the United States investigated the impact of the COVID-19 pandemic on HCV care by comparing the number of newly diagnosed patients during a three-month-period before COVID-19 measures with the subsequent three months. The authors found a 42% reduction in the number of new diagnoses [29]. To model the impact of COVID-19 on HCV elimination in The Netherlands, we assumed a similar decrease in diagnosis levels and furthermore assumed that the same decrease would also apply to the number of annually treated patients. In the third scenario (Two-year COVID-19 Delay), these reductions were assumed for 2020 and 2021, and model parameters were assumed to return to Status Quo values in 2022 and remain stable thereafter. The fourth scenario (Post-COVID Recovery Gradual Decline) assumed the same two-year delay in 2020–2021 and initial recovery in 2022, but furthermore assumed a continuous annual reduction of 10% in both newly diagnosed and treated patients from 2023 onwards. All model inputs for COVID-related scenarios can be found in Supplementary Tables S7 and S8.

3. Results

An estimated 11,327 patients were HCV-infected in 2016, of whom 3963 were estimated to be diagnosed. Following the Status Quo scenario of 630 new diagnoses and 698 treated patients annually, the WHO targets would be met by 2027 (Table 2). The incidence target, which was disregarded due to the extremely low pre-existing incidence in The Netherlands, would be met in 2034. In the Gradual Decline scenario, in which a yearly 10% reduction in diagnoses and treatments was implemented, WHO elimination targets would be met by 2032. The incidence target would not be met. All COVID-19-related scenario outcomes are detailed in Supplementary File S2, Figures S2 and S3, and Table S9. In general, an estimated 360 patients need to be treated annually from 2020–2030 in order to meet the treatment target by 2030.

Table 2. Forecasted year of elimination with scenarios "status quo" and "gradual decline".

WHO's Elimination Target	Year of Elimination	
	Status Quo	Gradual Decline
65% reduction in liver-related mortality	2020	2021
90% of infected patients diagnosed	2027	2032
80% of eligible patients treated	2025	2027
Year of elimination	2027	2032

All scenarios had a significant impact on the number of viraemic people (see Figure 1). The Status Quo scenario reduced viraemic HCV prevalence by 71% from 2015 to 2030, while the corresponding reduction in the Gradual Decline scenario was 50%. During the same time period, liver-related mortality was reduced by 97% in the Status Quo and 93% in the Gradual Decline scenario. Outcomes regarding liver-related morbidity and mortality are shown in Figure 2. The Gradual Decline scenario resulted in 12 excess cases of decompensated cirrhosis, 18 excess cases of hepatocellular carcinoma (HCC), and 20 excess cases of liver-related death from 2020–2030, compared to the Status Quo scenario.

The sensitivity analysis showed that a 15% reduction in annual diagnoses and treatments, as opposed to the 10% implemented in the Gradual Decline scenario, pushed back the WHO elimination targets significantly (see Table 3). The incidence target was not met, comparable to the Gradual Decline scenario. Furthermore, after an initial decrease, HCV prevalence started increasing from 2028 onward. The difference in liver-related morbidity and mortality was small, with one excess case of decompensated cirrhosis, two excess cases of hepatocellular carcinoma, and one excess case of liver-related death from 2020–2030, compared to the Gradual Decline scenario.

Table 3. Forecasted year of elimination in the sensitivity analysis.

WHO's Elimination Target	Year of Elimination
65% reduction in liver-related mortality	2021
90% of infected patients diagnosed	>2050
80% of eligible patients treated	2030
Year of elimination	**>2050**

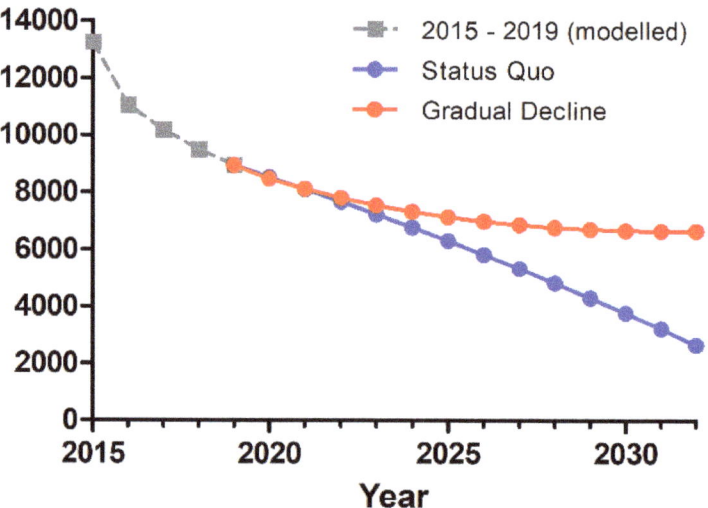

Figure 1. Predicted number of HCV-viraemic individuals in The Netherlands over time, following the Status Quo and Gradual Decline scenarios. HCV: hepatitis C virus.

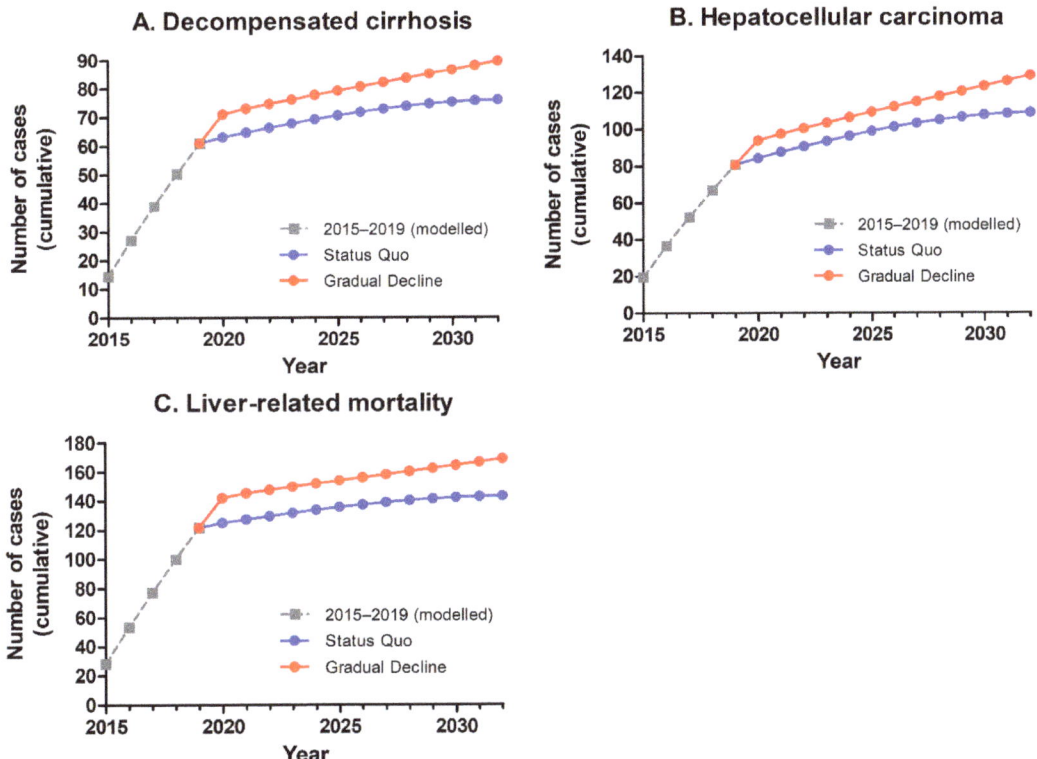

Figure 2. Predicted incident cases (cumulative) of (**A**) decompensated cirrhosis, (**B**) hepatocellular carcinoma, and (**C**) liver-related mortality in The Netherlands over time, following the Status Quo and Gradual Decline scenarios.

4. Discussion

The aim of this study was to predict when The Netherlands will meet the WHO HCV elimination targets. The results show that The Netherlands is on track to eliminate hepatitis C by 2030, if annual diagnosis and treatment rates can be maintained at 2019 levels. When an annual decrease of 10% was implemented for both diagnosis and treatment levels from 2021 onwards, WHO elimination targets were met by 2032. Both scenarios had a significant impact on viraemic prevalence and liver-related morbidity and mortality. Interestingly, the absolute numbers of incident cases of decompensated cirrhosis, hepatocellular carcinoma, and liver-related mortality sharply dropped, starting in 2020. This might be explained by the history of the HCV epidemic in The Netherlands.

The HCV epidemic took off during the heroin crisis in the 1970s, resulting in a wave of HIV and HCV infections [21]. Injecting drug use continuously decreased from 1985 to 2015, and concordantly, HIV and HCV incidence also dropped [21]. After 2000, a shift in HCV incidence from PWID to MSM was seen [22,23]. HCV infection is likely detected early in MSM due to regular testing, and treatment uptake in this group is high [30]. HCV-related morbidity and mortality in diagnosed MSM is therefore low. As most PWID have been infected from 1970–1990, the resulting peak in morbidity and mortality has most likely passed. When DAAs became available in 2014–2015, treatment was only reserved for people with F3 or F4 fibrosis. Combined with the continuous use of DAA therapy for all patients over the next few years, this may have resulted in a sharp decline in liver-related morbidity and mortality, as shown by our results. However, these modelled results need to be validated using real-life data. Hopefully, the future national HCV registry, currently in its pilot phase, will provide accurate data on HCV-related epidemiology, morbidity, and mortality.

Our results are more favourable than those of a recent study which estimated that The Netherlands would meet HCV elimination targets by 2035 [5]. The authors concluded that both the 90% diagnosis coverage and the 80% treatment coverage would be the first targets to be met, in 2025, and that the 65% reduction in liver-related mortality would follow in 2035. Remarkably, our study contrasts with these results, which may have various explanations. First, the base case prevalence used in our study differed from previously published studies using this model. In the current study, we estimated the number of currently viraemic people by subtracting the number of cured patients from the ever-infected population, using a high-quality treatment database and the most recent prevalence estimate [16,17]. This led to a slightly lower base-case viraemic prevalence compared to other studies. Furthermore, due to the larger number of cured patients, it is likely that morbidity and mortality outcomes appeared more favourable compared to other studies that used different methods. A third reason, which explains the difference regarding the treatment target, is the timing of the performed studies. As shown in Supplementary Figure S1, treatment numbers peaked after the introduction of DAAs (2015–2016) but declined shortly thereafter (2017–2019). It is possible that other, earlier studies extrapolated treatment numbers from the "peak" period, leading to an overestimation of subsequent treatment levels.

In view of the current pandemic, we modelled two scenarios projecting the impact of COVID-19. Both scenarios assumed a 42% reduction to Status Quo 2020 levels of annual diagnoses and treatments for two years, recovering to the Status Quo 2020 level in 2022. This reduction was based on a recent study from the United States [29], as Dutch data at the time of execution of this study was lacking. However, a recently published study showed that Dutch HCV diagnoses in 2020 decreased by 43% as compared to 2019, and that the weekly relative reduction mirrored the weekly number of COVID-19 admissions [31]. Furthermore, recently published treatment data by the GIP database show that 505 people have been treated for HCV in 2020, corresponding to a 35% decrease as compared to 2019 [17]. These data support the robustness of the COVID-19 scenario inputs. In the first COVID-19 scenario, diagnosis and treatment rates were kept constant after initial recovery in 2022, whereas the second assumed a 10% annual reduction from 2023 onwards. Remarkably, both scenarios resulted in earlier elimination than the Gradual Decline scenario, mainly due to the 90% diagnosis coverage target. This can be explained by the higher absolute number of new diagnoses and treatments during 2020–2030 in both COVID-19 scenarios compared to the Gradual Decline scenario. However, the number of liver-related deaths is higher for the COVID-19 scenarios (17 and 19 additional deaths, respectively, compared to the Gradual Decline scenario), which is also reflected in the year in which the 65% reduction in liver-related mortality is reached (2022 in both COVID-19 scenarios, compared to 2021 in the Gradual Decline scenario). Furthermore, both COVID-19 scenarios resulted in more cases of decompensated cirrhosis and hepatocellular carcinoma, although absolute numbers remain small.

The sensitivity analysis emphasizes the lack of flexibility in maintaining annual diagnosis and treatment levels in a low-prevalence country such as The Netherlands. A 15% reduction in these levels, as opposed to the 10% reduction in the Gradual Decline scenario, immediately resulted in the diagnosis target becoming unattainable before 2050. A 20% reduction resulted in the treatment target to be unattainable as well (results not shown). Eventually, the sensitivity analysis even resulted in an increase in viraemic HCV prevalence. This analysis therefore emphasizes the need to maintain high diagnosis and treatment levels in the upcoming years. However, maintaining high diagnosis and treatment levels may prove challenging. Unpublished data from the nationwide retrieval project (CELINE) on annual new diagnoses show a continuous decrease in the number of new diagnoses over the last five years, and GIP database data on annually treated patients show a similar decrease. Groups in The Netherlands with the highest absolute number of (prior) chronic

HCV infections are first-generation migrants from endemic countries, PWID, and people who have no (identified) risk factor for HCV infection [16]. These groups are harder to reach compared to other HCV risk groups. Fortunately, there are stakeholders in The Netherlands that aim to improve HCV care for these groups. Migrant screening, decentralization of HCV care in addiction care (CAC), and screening of prisoners are items currently high on the agenda. These efforts are vital in order to eliminate hepatitis C as a public health threat in The Netherlands. However, more support from the government is needed to enable these efforts.

5. Strengths and Limitations

This is the first Dutch modelling study that estimates the timing of the WHO elimination targets. We incorporated the most recent, published data, as well as unpublished data that has been collected during an ongoing nationwide retrieval project (CELINE). This unpublished data has confirmed previously published data, supported expert opinion, and given new insights into the Dutch HCV epidemic, strengthening the current analysis. Four realistic scenarios were devised, resulting in a robust elimination timeline. However, this study also has several limitations.

The model is limited by the accuracy of its input parameters. Unfortunately, as country-specific data was often missing, certain assumptions had to be made. In addition, the model itself makes certain assumptions as well. The annual number of HCV drug users was approximated based on GIP database data, which incorporated various assumptions, especially for the pre-DAA era. It is possible that people have been counted more than once, due to timing of treatment, treatment duration, and possible re-treatment after initial failure or re-infection. Furthermore, the model assumes that the distribution of treatments runs concordant to the genotype distribution and is equal in all risk groups. In reality, some genotypes and/or key populations were less likely to be treated due to suboptimal treatment results or barriers to treatment. Lastly, the model does not account for different SVR percentages after re-treatment due to failure or re-infection. These assumptions may have resulted in an overestimation of the number of treated and thereby cured patients, resulting in an underestimation of viraemic prevalence. Hopefully, once the national HCV registry is established, more accurate data on epidemiology, treatment, and (long-term) clinical outcomes will be available.

6. Conclusions

In conclusion, The Netherlands appears to be on track to reach HCV elimination by 2030, though many challenges remain. This study demonstrates what it takes to meet the elimination targets in time, which might guide us in developing and implementing the (public) health policies that are needed. Dutch HCV elimination still needs invested stakeholders to maintain and, where necessary, improve the existing infrastructures regarding HCV care. These study results should be used as a base with which we can compare our actions in the future.

Supplementary Materials: The following are available online at https://www.mdpi.com/article/10.3390/jcm10194562/s1, File S1: Available treatments and SVR percentages in The Netherlands, File S2: COVID-19 scenario results, Table S1: Total number of annual HCV antiviral drug users in The Netherlands, Table S2: Approximation of the number of annual HCV antiviral drug users for HCV infection in The Netherlands, Table S3: Calculated genotype-dependant SVR percentages during the (pegylated) interferon era (2000–2014), Table S4: Status Quo scenario model inputs, Table S5: Gradual decline scenario model inputs, Table S6: Sensitivity analysis model inputs, Table S7: Two-year COVID-19 Delay model inputs, Table S8: Post-COVID Recovery Gradual Decline model inputs, Table S9: Forecasted year of elimination with scenarios "Two-year COVID-19 Delay" and "Post-COVID Recovery Gradual Decline", Figure S1: Actual (continuous line) and predicted (dotted lines) number of patients treated with direct acting antivirals, Figure S2: Predicted number of HCV-viraemic individuals in The Netherlands over time, following the Two-year COVID-19 Delay and Post-recovery Gradual Decline scenarios, Figure S3: Predicted incident cases (cumulative) of (A) decompensated cirrhosis, (B) hepatocellular carcinoma, and (C) liver-related mortality in The Netherlands over time, following the Two-year COVID-19 Delay and Post-recovery Gradual Decline scenarios.

Author Contributions: M.v.D., S.M.B., C.J.I., J.P.H.D. and R.J.d.K. were involved in the design of this study, the acquisitioning of the data, and the expert consensus meetings. M.v.D. performed the analyses. M.v.D., S.M.B. and C.J.I. interpreted the data. M.v.D. drafted the manuscript. S.M.B., C.J.I., W.-H.C., G.B., H.B., A.S.M.D., B.v.H., C.v.N., M.J.S., M.v.d.V., J.P.H.D. and R.J.d.K. revised the manuscript critically for important intellectual content. All authors have read and agreed to the published version of the manuscript.

Funding: This study was non-funded. The model has been provided by AbbVie and the Centre for Disease Analysis. AbbVie did not have any role in study design, data collection, management, analysis and/or interpretation. Data from the CELINE project has been used in this study. The CELINE project is supported with an unrestricted grant from Gilead Sciences. Gilead Sciences did not have any role in study design, data collection, management, analysis and/or interpretation.

Institutional Review Board Statement: As data used in the development of this model were publicly available or were already collected in other, previously approved studies, ethical approval from an institutional review board was not required for the execution of this study.

Informed Consent Statement: Not applicable.

Data Availability Statement: The data presented in this study are available on request from the corresponding author.

Acknowledgments: We would like to thank Anouk T. Urbanus and Irene K. Veldhuijzen from the National Institute for Public Health and the Environment, and Daniela K. van Santen from the Municipal Health Services Amsterdam for their participation in expert consensus meetings and the acquisitioning of data. Furthermore, we thank Ivane Gamkrelidze for his help in calibrating the model, performing the analyses and critically revising the manuscript.

Conflicts of Interest: M.v.D. declares that the Radboudumc, on behalf of M.v.D., received honoraria due to participation in advisory boards of Abbvie and Gilead. S.M.B. and C.J.I. have no conflicts of interest. W.-H.C. is an employee of AbbVie and may own stocks and/or stock options of the company. J.P.H.D. declares that the Radboudumc, on behalf of J.P.H.D., received honoraria or research grants from Novartis, Ipsen, Otsuka, Abbvie, and Gilead. J.P.H.D. served as consultant for Gilead and Abbvie, and in the last two years has been member of advisory boards of Otsuka, Norgine Gilead, Bristol-Myers Squibb (B.-M.S.), Janssen, and Abbvie. R.d.K. declares that the Erasmus University Medical Centre, on behalf of R.d.K., received honoraria for consulting/speaking from Gilead, Janssen, B.-M.S., Abbvie, Merck Sharp & Dohme and Roche and received research grants from Abbvie, Gilead, GlaxoSmithKline and Janssen.

References

1. World Health Organization. *Global Hepatitis Report*; World Health Organization: Geneva, Switzerland, 2017; ISBN 978-92-4-156545-5.
2. World Health Organization. *Global Health Sector Strategy on Viral Hepatitis, 2016–2021*; Document number: WHO/HIV/2016.06; World Health Organization: Geneva, Switzerland, 2016.
3. Nayagam, S.; Thursz, M.; Sicuri, E.; Conteh, L.; Wiktor, S.; Low-Beer, D.; Hallett, T. Requirements for global elimination of hepatitis B: A modelling study. *Lancet Infect. Dis.* **2016**, *16*, 1399–1408. [CrossRef]
4. Razavi, H.; Waked, I.; Sarrazin, C.; Myers, R.P.; Idilman, R.; Calinas, F.; Vogel, W.; Mendes Correa, M.C.; Hézode, C.; Lázaro, P.; et al. The present and future disease burden of hepatitis C virus (HCV) infection with today's treatment paradigm. *J. Viral Hepat.* **2014**, *21* (Suppl. 1), 34–59. [CrossRef]
5. Gamkrelidze, I.; Pawlotsky, J.; Lazarus, J.V.; Feld, J.J.; Zeuzem, S.; Bao, Y.; dos Santos, A.G.P.; Gonzalez, Y.S.; Razavi, H. Progress towards hepatitis C virus elimination in high-income countries: An updated analysis. *Liver Int.* **2021**, *41*, 456–463. [CrossRef]
6. Isfordink, C.J.; Brakenhoff, S.M.; van Dijk, M.; van der Valk, M.; de Knegt, R.J.; Arends, J.E.; Drenth, J.P. Hepatitis C elimination in the Netherlands (CELINE): Study protocol for nationwide retrieval of lost to follow-up patients with chronic hepatitis C. *BMJ Open Gastroenterol.* **2020**, *7*, e000396. [CrossRef]

7. Staritsky, L.E.; Van Aar, F.; Visser, M.; Op de Coul, E.L.M.; Heijne, J.C.M.; Götz, H.M.; Nielen, M.; van Sighem, A.I.; van Benthem, B.H.B. *Sexually Transmitted Infections in The Netherlands in 2019*; National Institute for Public Health and the Environment (RIVM): Bilthoven, The Netherlands, 2020; ISBN 978-90-6960-294-3.
8. Willemse, S.B.; Razavi-Shearer, D.; Zuure, F.R.; Veldhuijzen, I.K.; A Croes, E.; Van Der Meer, A.J.; Van Santen, D.K.; De Vree, J.M.; De Knegt, R.J.; Zaaijer, H.L.; et al. The estimated future disease burden of hepatitis C virus in the Netherlands with different treatment paradigms. *Neth. J. Med.* **2015**, *73*, 417–431. [PubMed]
9. Polaris Observatory HCV Collaborators. Global prevalence and genotype distribution of hepatitis C virus infection in 2015: A modelling study. *Lancet Gastroenterol. Hepatol.* **2017**, *2*, 161–176. [CrossRef]
10. Müllhaupt, B.; Bruggmann, P.; Bihl, F.; Blach, S.; Lavanchy, D.; Razavi, H.; Semela, D.; Negro, F. Modeling the Health and Economic Burden of Hepatitis C Virus in Switzerland. *PLoS ONE* **2015**, *10*, e0125214. [CrossRef] [PubMed]
11. Razavi, H.; Robbins, S.; Zeuzem, S.; Negro, F.; Buti, M.; Duberg, A.-S.; Roudot-Thoraval, F.; Craxi, A.; Manns, M.; Marinho, R.T.; et al. Hepatitis C virus prevalence and level of intervention required to achieve the WHO targets for elimination in the European Union by 2030: A modelling study. *Lancet Gastroenterol. Hepatol.* **2017**, *2*, 325–336. [CrossRef]
12. Kwon, J.A.; Dore, G.J.; Grebely, J.; Hajarizadeh, B.; Guy, R.; Cunningham, E.B.; Power, C.; Estes, C.; Razavi, H.; Richard, T.G. Australia on track to achieve WHO HCV elimination targets following rapid initial DAA treatment uptake: A modelling study. *J. Viral Hepat.* **2019**, *26*, 83–92. [CrossRef]
13. Binka, M.; Janjua, N.Z.; Grebely, J.; Estes, C.; Schanzer, D.; Kwon, J.A.; Shoukry, N.H.; Kwong, J.C.; Razavi, H.; Feld, J.J.; et al. Assessment of Treatment Strategies to Achieve Hepatitis C Elimination in Canada Using a Validated Model. *JAMA Netw. Open.* **2020**, *3*, e204192. [CrossRef]
14. Kondili, L.A.; Robbins, S.; Blach, S.; Gamkrelidze, I.; Zignego, A.L.; Brunetto, M.R.; Raimondo, G.; Taliani, G.; Iannone, A.; Francesco, P. Russo. Forecasting Hepatitis C liver disease burden on real-life data. Does the hidden iceberg matter to reach the elimination goals? *Liver Int.* **2018**, *38*, 2190–2198. [CrossRef]
15. World Population Prospects: The 2019 Revision [Internet]. 2019. Available online: https://population.un.org/wpp/ (accessed on 20 January 2021).
16. Koopsen, J.; van Steenbergen, J.E.; Richardus, J.H.; Prins, M.; Op de Coul, E.L.M.; Croes, E.A.; Heil, J.; Zuure, F.R.; Veldhuijzen, I.K. Chronic hepatitis B and C infections in The Netherlands: Estimated prevalence in risk groups and the general population. *Epidemiol. Infect.* **2019**, *147*, e147. [CrossRef] [PubMed]
17. GIP Database. Available online: https://www.gipdatabank.nl/ (accessed on 26 September 2020).
18. Lyerla, R.; Gouws, E.; García-Calleja, J.M.; Zaniewski, E. The 2005 Workbook: An improved tool for estimating HIV prevalence in countries with low level and concentrated epidemics. *Sex. Transm. Infect.* **2006**, *82* (Suppl. 3), iii31. [CrossRef] [PubMed]
19. Statistics Netherlands. Asylum, Migration and Integration File. Available online: https://www.cbs.nl/nl-nl/dossier/dossier-asiel-migratie-en-integratie/hoeveel-immigranten-komen-naar-nederland- (accessed on 25 September 2020).
20. Falla, A.M.; Ahmad, A.A.; Duffell, E.; Noori, T.; Veldhuijzen, I.K. Estimating the scale of chronic hepatitis C virus infection in the EU/EEA: A focus on migrants from anti-HCV endemic countries. *BMC Infect Dis.* **2018**, *18*, 42. [CrossRef] [PubMed]
21. van Santen, D.K.; Coutinho, R.A.; van den Hoek, A.; van Brussel, G.; Buster, M.; Prins, M. Lessons learned from the Amsterdam Cohort Studies among people who use drugs: A historical perspective. *Harm Reduct. J.* **2021**, *18*, 2. [CrossRef] [PubMed]
22. Van den Broek, I.V.F.; Van Aar, F.; Van Oeffelen, A.A.M.; Op de Coul, E.L.M.; Woestenberg, P.J.; Heijne, J.C.M.; den Daas, C.; Hofstraat, S.H.I.; Hoenderboom, B.M.; van Wees, D. *Sexually Transmitted Infections in The Netherlands in 2015*; National Institute for Public Health and the Environment (RIVM): Bilthoven, The Netherlands, 2016; ISBN 978-90-6960-284-4.
23. Smit, C.; Boyd, A.; A Rijnders, B.J.; van de Laar, T.J.W.; Leyten, E.M.; Bierman, W.F.; Brinkman, K.; A A Claassen, M.; Hollander, J.D.; Boerekamps, A.; et al. HCV micro-elimination in individuals with HIV in the Netherlands 4 years after universal access to direct-acting antivirals: A retrospective cohort study. *Lancet HIV* **2021**, *8*, e96–e105. [CrossRef]
24. Visser, M.; Van Aar, F.; Van Oeffelen, A.A.M.; Van den Broek, I.V.F.; Op de Coul, E.L.M.; Hofstraat, S.H.I.; Heijne, J.C.M.; den Daas, C.; Hoenderboom, B.M.; van Wees, D.A. *Sexually Transmitted Infections Including HIV, in The Netherlands in 2016*; National Institute for Public Health and the Environment (RIVM): Bilthoven, The Netherlands, 2017; ISBN 978-90-6960-287-5.
25. Polaris Observatory Collaborators. The case for simplifying and using absolute targets for viral hepatitis elimination goals. *J. Viral Hepat.* **2021**, *28*, 12–19. [CrossRef]
26. Hatzakis, A.; Chulanov, V.; Gadano, A.C.; Bergin, C.; Ben-Ari, Z.; Mossong, J.; Schréter, I.; Baatarkhuu, O.; Acharya, S.; Aho, I. The present and future disease burden of hepatitis C virus (HCV) infections with today's treatment paradigm-volume 2. *J. Viral Hepat.* **2015**, *22* (Suppl. 1), 26–45. [CrossRef]
27. Dinmohamed, A.G.; Visser, O.; Verhoeven, R.H.A.; Louwman, M.W.J.; van Nederveen, F.H.; Willems, S.M.; Merkx, M.A.W.; Lemmens, V.E.P.P.; Nagtegaal, I.D.; Siesling, S. Fewer cancer diagnoses during the COVID-19 epidemic in the Netherlands. *Lancet Oncol.* **2020**, *21*, 750–751. [CrossRef]
28. de Vries, A.P.J.; Alwayn, I.P.J.; Hoek, R.A.S.; van den Berg, A.P.; Ultee, F.C.W.; Vogelaar, S.M.; Haase-Kromwijk, B.J.J.M.; Heemskerk, M.B.A.; Hemke, A.C.; Nijboer, W.N. Immediate impact of COVID-19 on transplant activity in the Netherlands. *Transpl. Immunol.* **2020**, *61*, 101304. [CrossRef] [PubMed]
29. Sperring, H.; Ruiz-Mercado, G.; Schechter-Perkins, E.M. Impact of the 2020 COVID-19 Pandemic on Ambulatory Hepatitis C Testing. *J. Prim. Care Community Health* **2020**. [CrossRef] [PubMed]

30. Boerekamps, A.; Newsum, A.M.; Smit, C.; Arends, J.E.; Richter, C.; Reiss, P.; Rijnders, B.J.A.; Brinkman, K.; van der Valk, M. High Treatment Uptake in Human Immunodeficiency Virus/Hepatitis C Virus-Coinfected Patients After Unrestricted Access to Direct-Acting Antivirals in the Netherlands. *Clin. Infect. Dis.* **2018**, *66*, 1352–1359. [CrossRef] [PubMed]
31. Sonneveld, M.J.; Veldhuijzen, I.K.; van de Laar, T.; Op de Coul, E.L.M.; van der Meer, A.J. Decrease in viral hepatitis diagnoses during the COVID-19 pandemic in the Netherlands. *J. Hepatol.* **2021**. Online ahead of print. [CrossRef] [PubMed]

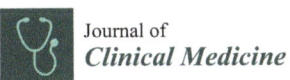 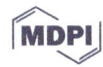

Article

Out-of-Hospital Treatment of Hepatitis C Increases Retention in Care among People Who Inject Drugs and Homeless Persons: An Observational Study

Bianca Granozzi [1], Viola Guardigni [1,*], Lorenzo Badia [1], Elena Rosselli Del Turco [1], Alberto Zuppiroli [1], Beatrice Tazza [1], Pietro Malosso [1], Stefano Pieralli [2], Pierluigi Viale [1] and Gabriella Verucchi [1]

1 Infectious Diseases Unit, Department of Medical and Surgical Sciences, University of Bologna, 40139 Bologna, Italy; bianca.granozzi@gmail.com (B.G.); lorenzo.badia@aosp.bo.it (L.B.); erossellidelturco@gmail.com (E.R.D.T.); alberto.zuppiroli@studio.unibo.it (A.Z.); bea.tazza@gmail.com (B.T.); pietro.malosso@gmail.com (P.M.); pierluigi.viale@unibo.it (P.V.); gabriella.verucchi@unibo.it (G.V.)
2 Open Group Society Coop. Soc. Onlus, 40139 Bologna, Italy; pierallis@gmail.com
* Correspondence: v.guardigni@gmail.com; Tel.: +39-333-4502053

Citation: Granozzi, B.; Guardigni, V.; Badia, L.; Rosselli Del Turco, E.; Zuppiroli, A.; Tazza, B.; Malosso, P.; Pieralli, S.; Viale, P.; Verucchi, G. Out-of-Hospital Treatment of Hepatitis C Increases Retention in Care among People Who Inject Drugs and Homeless Persons: An Observational Study. *J. Clin. Med.* **2021**, *10*, 4955. https://doi.org/10.3390/jcm10214955

Academic Editors: Maria Carla Liberto and Nadia Marascio

Received: 9 October 2021
Accepted: 21 October 2021
Published: 26 October 2021

Publisher's Note: MDPI stays neutral with regard to jurisdictional claims in published maps and institutional affiliations.

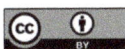

Copyright: © 2021 by the authors. Licensee MDPI, Basel, Switzerland. This article is an open access article distributed under the terms and conditions of the Creative Commons Attribution (CC BY) license (https://creativecommons.org/licenses/by/4.0/).

Abstract: Background. People who inject drugs (PWID) and homeless people represent now a large reservoir of Hepatitis C virus (HCV) infection. However, Hepatis C elimination programs can barely reach these subgroups of patients. We aimed to evaluate and compare the retention in care among these difficult-to-treat patients when managed for HCV in hospital or in an out-of-hospital setting. Methods. In our retrospective study, we categorized the included patients (PWID and homeless persons) into two groups according to whether anti-HCV treatment was offered and provided in a hospital or an out-of-hospital setting. We run logistic regressions to evaluate factors associated with retention in care (defined as the completion of direct antiviral agents (DAAs) therapy). Results. We included 56 patients in our study: 27 were in the out-of-hospital group. Overall, 33 patients completed DAAs therapy. A higher rate of retention in care was observed in the out-of-hospital group rather than in-hospital group ($p = 0.001$). At the univariate analysis, retention in care was associated with the out-of-hospital management ($p = 0.002$) and with a shorter time between the first visit and the scheduled start of DAAs ($p = 0.003$). Conclusions. The choice of treatment models that can better adapt to difficult-to-treat populations, such as an out-of-hospital approach, will be important for achieving the eradication of HCV infection.

Keywords: PWID; homeless persons; HCV eradication; direct-acting antivirals; out-of-hospital; retention in care

1. Introduction

The worldwide incidence and prevalence of Hepatitis C virus (HCV) infection has been decreasing since the introduction of the new direct antiviral agents (DAAs) as a form of standard of care [1,2] and the World Health Organization (WHO) has established the global goal of eradicating hepatitis C infection as a public health threat by 2030 [3].

Currently, injection drug use represents the primary route of transmission of HCV infection and the main viral reservoir consists of people who inject drugs (PWID) [4,5], among whom a global anti-HCV seroprevalence of 52.3% has been estimated [6].

Prevalence studies have reported that also homeless persons are at high risk for HCV, mostly as a result of injection drug use [7]. Indeed, PWID tend to experience homelessness or unstable housing with prevalence ranging from 6.7% in Eastern Europe to 50.3% in North America [6].

Homelessness and unstable housing have been recently associated to a greater risk for acquiring infections such as HCV and human immunodeficiency virus (HIV) among PWID when compared to PWID who had stable house [8]. A large meta-analysis has estimated an overall prevalence of HCV infection ranged from 3.9% to 36.2% in homeless people, based on the results of 12 eligible studies [7]. However, there is a scarcity of epidemiological data on the real prevalence of HCV infection in these difficult to treat subgroups [5]. Since HCV elimination programs barely reach these populations, targeted screening programs are necessary to achieve the goal set by the WHO [4]. For a long time, PWID has been regarded as a neglected population due to the concerns about adherence to treatments and poor treatment outcome. Among others, the MISTRAL study has shown how a safe and effective pan-genotypic treatment regimen, particularly with a short duration, could facilitate an increase in accessing treatments for high-risk populations [9,10]. Currently, guidelines for hepatitis C treatment from both the American and the European Association for the Study of Liver Diseases recommends to treat PWID with chronic HCV infection [11,12].

Factors complicating access to care in this population must be addressed including the stigma, the risk for reinfection in PWID, challenges related to incarceration, and housing instability [5,13].

It is also widely recognized that an integrated harm reduction strategy is needed to control HCV transmission and to reduce community viral load [6,14]. By reducing risk behaviors, HCV testing programs that combine screening and counseling can decrease HCV transmission and reinfection after treatment with DAAs [15,16]. The provision of sterile injecting equipment through needle and syringe programs and the enrolment in opioid substitution treatment (OST) are among the primary interventions for reducing HCV reinfection rate among PWID [17].

Recent data have shown that the incidence of HCV reinfections in PWID after achieving sustained viral response (SVR) is low (1.85–22.32/1000 person-years), with higher rates in active drug users [18,19].

Screening and confirmation tests, linkage to care, retention in care, prescription of DAAs, and adherence to HCV treatment are priorities for fighting the silent epidemic of chronic HCV infection in PWID and homeless people [9,20].

However, PWID and homeless persons have poor access to hospital care due to reduced retention in care and difficulties in accessing traditional screening programs. Therefore, alternative treatment approaches for PWID and homeless people are emerging across Europe [17,20–23].

In Italy, out-of-hospital care models are emerging with the presence of dedicated doctors, nurses, and peer-educators with experience in drug addiction [24–26]. In Italy, the "Stop HCV" project was conceived and conducted in the city of Bologna with the help of the "Open Group-Unità di Strada", a non-profit organization of harm reduction. The project consisted in offering HCV screening and treatment for hepatitis C using DOT (directly observed therapy), in a population of PWID and homeless people, with this occurring in an out-of-hospital setting.

The primary aim of our retrospective study was to measure and compare the retention in care rate, (defined as the completion of DAAs therapy) achieved in a group consisting of PWID and/or homeless persons with hepatitis C managed in a traditional hospital setting (i.e., outpatient services) with the retention in care rate achieved in a group of PWID and/or homeless persons but managed in an out-of-hospital setting.

The secondary aim of the study was to estimate prevalence of patients who started treatment after their linkage-to-care, the time between first visit and the scheduled start of therapy (defined as expected waiting time), and the rate of sustained virological response 12 weeks after the end of treatment (SVR 12).

2. Materials and Methods

We carried out a retrospective observational study including patients with HCV chronic infection (i.e., with documented detectable HCV RNA), considered eligible for DAAs treatment, who were active or past intravenous drug users and/or who were experiencing homelessness. In order to test our hypothesis that an out-of-hospital setting might ensure a greater retention in care in difficult-to-treat populations, we compared our outcomes between patients with similar characteristics but treated for HCV in different circumstances (i.e., out-of-hospital and in-hospital services).

Therefore, we included in the study all the patients with confirmed current HCV infection and history of injection drug use or homelessness who access the out-of-hospital facility where "Senza la C" project was established from January to June 2019.

This outpatient care model included an initial screening for HCV using saliva rapid tests (OraQuick® Rapid HCV Antibody by OraSure Technologies, Bethlehem, PA, USA) and a pre-test peer counseling offered by educators from Open Group Onlus, the community-based service for harm reduction we mentioned beforehand. Patients also received face-to-face counselling on HCV treatment, prevention, and re-infection risk.

In case of reactive saliva HCV-Ab test, a point of care HCV-RNA test on whole blood (Xpert® HCV VL Fingerstick by Cepheid, Sunnyvale, CA, USA), transient elastography (Fibroscan® by Echosens, Paris, France) and liver ultrasound were performed. Those who resulted HCV-RNA positive were tested through standard blood tests for liver and kidney function and HCV genotype and they were scheduled to start HCV treatment within three to four weeks.

Each of the following visits was conducted at DAAs initiation, after 4 weeks, at the end of therapy, and 12 weeks and 24 weeks after the end of therapy. HCV RNA viremia was performed at each visit in order to rule out any possible relapse or reinfection.

All diagnostic procedures, drug supplying, treatment monitoring, and post-treatment follow-up were conducted in a low-threshold, extra hospital setting by a team of peer educators, medical doctors, and trained nurses.

We considered as a comparison, a group of patients who met the inclusion criteria and with demographics (age and sex) similar to the group of interest, who had referred to a traditional hospital setting for a visit from May 2017 to August 2018 at our clinic of Infectious Diseases in Bologna (Italy), and were invited by clinicians to start DAAs treatment.

In the out-of-hospital setting, DOT (under the supervision of medical and not-medical staff) was applied, with the support of peer-educators with expertise in management of PWID, in the context of the "Stop HCV" project, which we have already mentioned.

All of the patients included in the study who started anti-HCV treatment, received DAAs for 8 or 12 weeks, according to international guidelines.

We assessed retention in care, defined as the completion of the established DAAs therapy, among our study population. We also measured the expected waiting time, which was defined as the time between the first visit and the scheduled start of therapy with DAAs. With regard to the proportion of population who started and completed treatment for hepatitis C, we observed them for six months after end of treatment. For each subject, we collected the following data at baseline: demographics (age, sex, BMI), stage of liver fibrosis (measured by transient elastography, FibroScan® by Echosens, Paris, France), prior failures to anti-HCV treatment, HCV genotype, HCV RNA viremia, DAAs regimen, data on HIV coinfection when present (i.e., HIV RNA viremia, CD4+T-cells count, current antiretroviral regimen), HBV coinfection (i.e., HBsAg positivity), psychiatric comorbidity, OST, and drug use status (i.e., current PWID or not). INR, bilirubin level, ALT level, creatinine level, and HCV RNA viremia were then evaluated at each scheduled visit.

Statistical Analysis

Patient characteristics were expressed as median (and Interquartile range, IQR) and percentage when appropriate. The normality of data distribution was assessed with the Shapiro–Wilk test. To compare the characteristics between groups (i.e., in hospital and out-of-hospital setting), we performed the Mann–Whitney U-test and the Chi-squared test (or Fisher Test when appropriate) for continuous and categorical variables, respectively. A p-value < 0.05 was considered statistically significant. To evaluate the variables associated with our primary outcome (i.e., retention in care) we performed logistic regression analysis, including in the multivariable model variables which presented a p-value ≤ 0.1 at univariate analysis. All of the analyses were performed by using IBM SPSS Statistics for (Windows, Version 24.0, Armonk, NY, USA).

3. Results

3.1. Patient Characteristics at Baseline

We enrolled 56 patients who met the inclusion criteria: this included 29 subjects in the in-hospital group and 27 subjects in the out-of-hospital group (as shown in Figure 1). The baseline characteristics are shown in Table 1. The median age was 44.5 years and 92.9% of patients were male. All the subjects in the in-hospital group actively used drugs at enrollment, while only 44.4% of those in the out-of-hospital were PWID ($p < 0.001$). Eleven out of 27 patients referring to out-of-hospital service were experiencing homelessness, whereas only one patient (a 51 years-old female) within the in-hospital setting was homeless, at the time of study participation. All of the patients included in this study had a positive history of intravenous drug use (current or previus).

Table 1. Baseline patients' characteristics, represented for total population and sorted by in-hospital and out-of-hospital setting where chronic hepatitis C was managed.

Characteristics	Total Population (n = 56)	In-Hospital Group (n = 29)	Out-of-Hospital Group (n = 27)	p Value
Age (year), median (IQR)	44.5 (35.5–51)	45 (36.5–50.5)	41 (35.0–51)	0.941
Male, n (%)	52.0 (92.9%)	27 (93.1%)	25 (92.6%)	1.000
BMI, median (IQR)	22.8 (20.8–24.8)	23.2 (21.0–27.2)	22.6 (20.1–24.5)	0.154
Active PWID	41 (73.2%)	29 (100%)	12 (44.4%)	<0.001
Previous PWID	15 (26.8%)	0 (0%)	15 (55.6%)	0.001
Homeless	12 (21.4%)	1 (3.4%)	11 (40.7%)	0.001
OST, n (%)	40.0 (71.4%)	26.0 (89.7%)	14.0 (51.9%)	0.003
Psychiatric comorbidity, n (%)	15.0 (26.8%)	6.0 (20.7%)	9.0 (33.3%)	0.370
HBsAg positive, n (%)	1.0 (1.9%)	1 (3.4%)	0.0 (0.0%)	1.000
HIV coinfection, n (%)	13.0 (24.5%)	10.0 (34.5%)	3.0 (12.5%)	0.108
Liver Stiffness [1], kPa, median (IQR)	6.5 (5.1–8.2)	6.8 (5.1–8.6)	6.35 (5.0–8.1)	0.434
Child-Pugh class [2], n (%)				
A	6	3	3	1
B	2	1	1	
HCV genotype, n (%)				
1	30.0 (58.8%)	14.0 (53.8%)	16.0 (64%)	
3	16.0 (31.4%)	9.0 (34.6%)	7.0 (28%)	0.754
4	5.0 (9.8%)	3.0 (11.5%)	2.0 (8%)	
Prior Peg-IFN/RBV failure, n (%)	8.9 (14.8%)	2.0 (7.4%)	6.0 (22.2%)	0.250
HCV RNA, $\log_{10}$ IU/mL, median (IQR)	6.1 (5.2–6.3)	6.1 (5.4–6.4)	6.0 (5.0–6.3)	0.741
ALT, IU/L, median (IQR)	45.0 (29.0–110)	44.0 (28.3–110)	55.0 (30.0–110)	0.899
Total bilirubin, mg/dL, median (IQR)	0.6 (0.4–0.8)	0.6 (0.4–0.9)	0.6 (0.4–0.8)	0.381
Creatinine, mg/dL, median (IQR)	0.8 (0.7–0.9)	0.9 (0.8–1)	0.7 (0.6–0.8)	0.003
Platelets, $\times 10^9$/L, median (IQR)	218 (177–266)	202 (152–253)	234 (185–273)	0.108

[1] assessed by transient elastography (FibroScan®), [2] variable described only for those patients with documented diagnosis of liver cirrhosis (n = 8). Abbreviations: BMI, body mass index; PWID, people who inject drugs; OST, opioid substitute therapy; IFN, interferon; RBV, ribavirin.

An overall of 71.4% of individuals (40/56) used OST, with a lower percentage in the out-of-hospital setting rather than the comparison setting (p = 0.003). Psychiatric comorbidity was found in 26.8% (15/56) of patients; 58.8% (30/56) of subjects were infected with HCV genotype 1. Five out of fifty-six patients (8.9%) had F3 fibrosis according to Metavir score, while 15.7% (8/56) had documented liver cirrhosis: two out of these eight subjects with an advanced liver disease had decompensated cirrhosis (B8 Child-Pugh class). There was a statistically significant difference in creatinine values between the two groups, with higher levels among those who were treated in the standard in-hospital setting (p = 0.003). Thirteen patients (24,5%) were HCV-HIV coinfected: characteristics of this particular subset of patients are shown in Table 2.

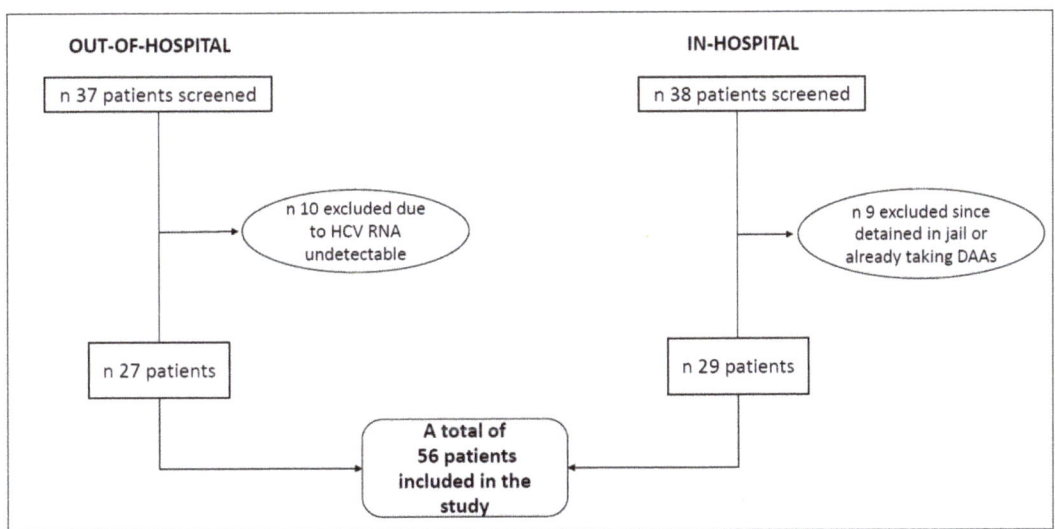

Figure 1. Flow chart of study enrollment.

Table 2. Patients with HIV/HCV coinfection.

Parameters	Total Population (*n* = 13)	In-Hospital Group (*n* = 10)	Out-of-Hospital Group (*n* = 3)	*p* Value
Undetectable HIV RNA, *n* (%)	9 (75%)	8 (88.9%)	1 (33.3%)	0.127
CD4+ cell count/mm^3, median (IQR)	632 (419–849)	575 (377–891)	688 (545–746)	1.000
ART regimen, *n* (%)				
2NRTI + NNRTI	4 (33.3%)	3 (33.3%)	1 (33.3%)	
2NRTI + INSTI	3 (25%)	2 (22.2%)	1 (33.3%)	0.931
2NRTI + PI	1 (8.3%)	1 (11.1%)	none	
Others	4 (33.3%)	3 (33.3%)	1 (33.3%)	

Abbreviation: ART, antiretroviral therapy; NRTI, nucleoside reverse transcriptase inhibitors; NNRTI, non-nucleoside reverse transcriptase inhibitors; INSTI, integrase strand transfer inhibitors; PI, protease inhibitors.

3.2. Primary and Secondary Outcomes

In our study population, 33 out of 56 patients started therapy with DAAs. The most used HCV regimen was Glecaprevir/Pibrentasvir (73% treated for 8 weeks, 9% for 12 weeks). The remaining patients received therapy with Sofosbuvir/Velpatasvir. All of the 33 patients who started DAAs (corresponding to 60% of the study population) completed treatment with DAAs, with no difference between groups. However, when we analyzed the rate of retention in care (defined as DAAs treatment start and completion, as described in Section 2) among the total study population (56 patients), we observed a higher rate of retention in care in the out-of-hospital group than in standard in-hospital setting (p = 0.001), Figure 2A. The expected waiting time was significantly longer in subjects referring to standard in-hospital services (p < 0.001), in comparison with the other group (Figure 2B). Among the 33 patients who were treated for Hepatitis C, 93.9% achieved SVR 12 (31/33), with similar SVR12 rates among the two groups (Table 3). The two patients (one in each of the two groups) did not achieve sustained virological response: one experienced a relapse after four weeks from the end of treatment (in-hospital group) and one was diagnosed with HCV reinfection over the follow-up (out-of-hospital group). At the univariate analysis, retention in care was associated only with the out-of-hospital management (p = 0.002) and with a shorter expected waiting time (p = 0.003), as shown in Table 4. At the multivariate analysis, when we included the covariate "expected waiting time" in the model with "out-of-hospital management" as an exposure variable, the out-of-hospital management did not remain statistically significant as a predictor of retention in care (O.R. 099, $p = 0.69$), while the "expected waiting time" showed a definite trend for association with retention in care, although not still significant (O.R. 0.65, $p = 0.08$). This could potentially suggest that our primary outcome (i.e., retention in care) might be driven by a shorter expected waiting time rather than the setting where patients were managed. When we analyzed the association of parameters with retention in care considering only the 41 patients who were actively using intravenous drugs at time of enrollment, we found that a greater retention in care rate was achieved among those treated out of the hospital (58%) than in the hospital (38%), although not statistically significant ($p = 0.31$). At the univariate analysis, we did not observe any variable associated with our primary outcome, although a shorter waiting time seemed to suggest a higher chance to complete DAAs therapy (Exp (B) 0.995, CI 95% 0.99;1, $p = 0.055$).

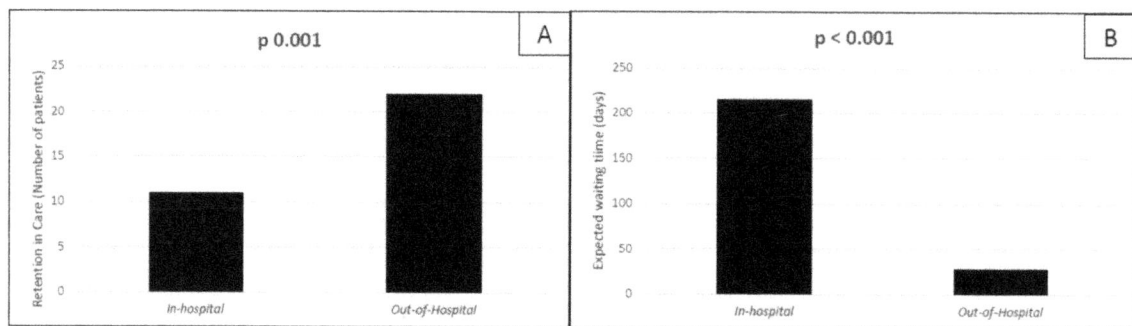

Figure 2. Patients treated with DAAs in our population. Retention in care rates among patients treated for HCV in hospital and out of hospital Panel (**A**); expected days of waiting before DAAs treatment start in the standard in-hospital setting group and in the out-of-hospital setting group panel (**B**).

Table 3. Comparison of primary and secondary outcomes between in-hospital and out-of-hospital settings.

Outcomes	Total Population ($n = 56$)	In-Hospital Group ($n = 29$)	Out-of-Hospital Group ($n = 27$)	p Value
Retention in care [1], n (%)	33 (58.9%)	11 (37.9%)	22 (81.5%)	0.001
Expected waiting time [2], days, median (IQR)	42 (28.0–215.3)	216 (168.5–314.8)	28.0 (21.0–28.0)	<0.001
SVR12, n (%)	Treated population ($n = 33$) 31 (93.9%)	In-hospital group ($n = 11$) 10 (90.9%)	Out-of-hospital group ($n = 22$) 21 (94.5%)	0.6

[1] completion of DAAs treatment; [2] time between the first medical visit and the scheduled DAAs treatment initiation. Abbreviation: SVR12, sustained virological response 12 weeks after end of treatment.

Overall, 37 patients accessed the established out-of-hospital service from January through June 2019 and were all screened for the study. All of them were past or current intravenous drug users or homeless persons. For the comparison group, we considered all the intravenous drug users with detectable HCV RNA who accessed traditional in-hospital service for a visit from May 2017 through August 2018, and we screened a total of 38 patients.

Table 4. Univariate analysis of factors associated to the retention in care.

Variables	Univariate Analysis		
	Exp (B)	95% CI	p-Value
Age	1.042	0.989; 1.099	0.123
Male sex	0.68	0.088; 5.19	0.71
Metavir F4	0.281	0.031; 2.552	0.26
BMI	0.91	0.79; 1.047	0.18
Homelessness	1.032	0.28; 3.77	0.96
OST	2.71	0.747; 9.87	0.129
Psychiatric comorbidity	0.64	0.19; 2.2	0.48
HIV coinfection	1.43	0.40; 5.1	0.58
Prior Peg-IFN/RBV failure	3.13	0.66; 14.8	0.15
ALT	1.002	0.99; 1.01	0.71
Bilirubin	1.25	0.453; 3.46	0.67
Creatinine	0.128	0.006; 2.77	0.19
Platelets	0.997	0.99; 1.004	0.434
Expected waiting time [1], days	0.992	0.987; 0.997	0.003
Out-of-hospital management	0.139	0.041; 0.474	0.002

[1] time between the first medical visit and the scheduled DAAs treatment initiation. Abbreviations: BMI, body mass index; OST, opioid substitute therapy; IFN, interferon; RBV, ribavirin.

4. Discussion

HCV infection is efficiently spread by injection drug use, and this represents an important public health issue. Furthermore, PWID are very challenging patients to treat due to their difficulties in accessing traditional care in hospital settings and the frequent co-occurrence of alcohol abuse, HIV infection, and psychiatric comorbidities [5,6]. Due to the difficulties in treating PWID, along with often asymptomatic course of HCV infection, there is a risk of underestimating individuals affected by hepatitis C [1]. Similarly, hepatitis C infection represents one of the most prevalent infectious disease among homeless people, and therefore they should be considered a high-risk group and for whom diagnosis and treatment of HCV should be a priority [7]. This lack of data on the real prevalence of HCV infection limits the WHO's goal of eradicating hepatitis C around the world [2]. Attempts to associate harm reduction interventions simultaneously with the administration of safe and short therapeutic regimens may favor a lowered transmission of the virus and a reduction of liver damage in these populations [9,10]. For these reasons, alternative models of care in out-of-hospital setting are spreading in Europe and Italy, with encouraging results [24–26]. Our study showed how an out-of-hospital care model might guarantee a greater percentage of patients starting DAAs with an overall better retention in care for difficult-to-reach groups with HCV infection. In our population, the patients with diagnosis of chronic hepatitis C managed in the out-of-hospital setting were more likely to initiate and complete the therapy, achieving the primary outcome, in comparison to the individuals treated in hospital ($p = 0.002$). Consistently with that, those who were scheduled to start a treatment with DAAs earlier after their first visit were more likely to complete the treatment for HCV infection than those who had to start DAAs with delay ($p = 0.003$). The significantly longer waiting time between the first access to hospital and the scheduled therapy initiation in comparison to the waiting time in out-of-hospital services (216 vs. 28 days) could have represented the major barrier to the "in-hospital" treatment and could explain the lower rate of DAAs treatment in this specific group. All the patients who started therapy were able to complete it (33/33). Therefore, treatment, per se, did not represent an obstacle in completing DAAs therapy in our population. A shorter expected waiting time seemed to increase the retention in care in active PWID (as anticipated). Also, when we focused our analysis on this specific subset of study population (although not statistically significant). We can reasonably assume from our analysis and results that a shorter waiting time is the key for the success of out-of-hospital approach, suggesting that it may play a role as a mediator for a higher proportion of retention in care in the out-of-hospital setting. Moreover, the presence of peer educators may have contributed to improve the linkage to care in the out-of-hospital setting. Starting treatment quickly and in a more individualized way improved the retention in care of PWID [17,20,24,26]. In agreement with our findings, recent research conducted in Vienna on DAAs administration as DOT (given at OST facilities) in PWID showed excellent SVR12 rates (99%) in this difficult-to-treat population, similar to patients with expected high treatment compliance in a standard setting [27]. In our study, although the rate of DAAs therapy completion was lower among patients treated in hospital, when we consider the entire subset of subjects who completed treatment, we observed similarly high virological success rates regardless from treatment setting with no statistically significant differences. The 93.9% of SVR 12 in our overall treated population confirmed the efficacy of regimens with DAAs as reported in the real-world published studies [28]. Small sample size and its retrospective nature are limitations of the study. Moreover, this is a real-world study and we have to acknowledge some baseline differences between the two groups that we compared in the analysis. In particular, all of the patients in the in-hospital group were active intravenous drug users, while less than 50% of the out-of-hospital group was currently using intravenous drugs: for this reason, we ran the same analysis including only active PWID. The presence of educators with expertise in the management of PWID, which are usually lacking in a traditional hospital setting, might also have contributed to the better retention in care achieved in the out-of-hospital facility. In addition, the "Stop HCV project" was interrupted due to a lack of funds. A prolongation of this program would have added relevant data, such as reinfection rate. The results of an effective anti-HCV treatment can be compromised by the risk of reinfection, associated with the persistence of risk behaviors after achieving SVR. For this reason, for a long time, PWID has been regarded as a neglected. However, recent published data have showed how the incidence of HCV reinfection in PWID after the achievement of SVR is low (1.85 to 22.32/1000 person-years) [18,29]. Longer follow-up periods could have certainly provided further data on this population.

In conclusions, our study demonstrated that underserved patients with chronic hepatitis C, historically defined as "difficult-to-treat" groups due to their social instability and risky behaviors, might benefit from new integrated healthcare approaches, such as an out-of-hospital setting where patients may be diagnosed with chronic HCV infection and cured shortly afterwards. The choice of treatment models that can better adapt to difficult populations, such as PWID and homeless people, will be important for achieving the WHO's goal and therefore further studies are needed.

Author Contributions: Conceptualization, B.G. and V.G.; methodology, V.G.; software, V.G.; investigation, B.G., L.B., B.T., S.P. and P.M.; data curation, V.G. and A.Z.; writing—original draft preparation, B.G.; writing—review and editing, V.G. and E.R.D.T.; supervision, G.V. and P.V.; project administration, L.B.; funding acquisition, P.V., L.B. and G.V. All authors have read and agreed to the published version of the manuscript.

Funding: This research was funded by Gilead Sciences (Fellowship Program/Digital Health Program 2018), grant number 04284.

Institutional Review Board Statement: The study was conducted according to the guidelines of Declaration of Helsinki, and approved by the Ethics Committee of Policlinico S. Orsola-Malpighi in Bologna (Italy), with the code CE 663/2019/Oss/AOUBo (date 20 November 2019).

Informed Consent Statement: Informed consent was obtained from all subjects involved in the study.

Data Availability Statement: The data that support the findings of this study are available from the corresponding author, (VG), upon reasonable request.

Acknowledgments: We thank Gilead Sciences that supported this work by Gilead Fellowship Program 2018.

Conflicts of Interest: The authors declare no conflict of interest. The funders had no role in the design of the study; in the collection, analyses, or interpretation of data; in the writing of the manuscript; or in the decision to publish the results.

References

1. WHO. Global Hepatitis Report 2017: Web Annex B: WHO Estimates of the Prevalence and Incidence of Hepatitis C Virus Infection by WHO Region, 2015. 2018. Available online: https://apps.who.int/iris/bitstream/handle/10665/277005/WHO-CDS-HIV-18.46-eng.pdf (accessed on 9 October 2021).
2. WHO. Global Report on Access to Hepatitis C Treatment—Focus on Overcoming Barriers. Available online: http://www.who.int/Hepatitis/publications/hep-c-access-report/en/ (accessed on 10 October 2021).
3. WHO Website. Available online: https://www.who.int/news-room/fact-sheets/detail/hepatitis-c (accessed on 10 October 2021).
4. Centers for Disease Control and Prevention (CDC). Division of Viral Hepatitis 2025 Strategic Plan, CDC. Available online: https://www.hhs.gov/hepatitis/viral-hepatitis-national-strategic-plan/index.html (accessed on 25 October 2021).
5. Schillie, S.; Wester, C. CDC Recommendations for Hepatitis C Screening Among Adults—United States, 2020. *MMWR Recomm. Rep.* **2020**, *69*, 1–17. [CrossRef] [PubMed]
6. Degenhardt, L.; Peacock, A. Global prevalence of injecting drug use and sociodemographic characteristics and prevalence of HIV, HBV, and HCV in people who inject drugs: A multistage systematic review. *Lancet Glob. Health* **2017**, *5*, e1192–e1207. [CrossRef]
7. Beijer, U.; Wolf, A. Prevalence of tuberculosis, Hepatitis C virus, and HIV in homeless people: A systematic review and meta-analysis. *Lancet Infect. Dis.* **2012**, *12*, 859–870. [CrossRef] [PubMed]
8. Arum, C.; Fraser, H. Homelessness, HIV, and HCV Review Collaborative Group. Homelessness, unstable housing, and risk of HIV and Hepatitis C virus acquisition among people who inject drugs: A systematic review and meta-analysis. *Lancet Public Health* **2021**, *6*, e309–e323. [CrossRef] [PubMed]
9. Persico, M.; Aglitti, A. Real-life glecaprevir/pibrentasvir in a large cohort of patients with Hepatitis C virus infection: The MISTRAL study. *Liver Int.* **2019**, *39*, 1852–1859. [CrossRef]
10. Foster, G.R.; Dore, G. Glecaprevir/pibrentasvir in patients with chronic HCV and recent drug use: An integrated analysis of 7 phase III studies. *Drug Alcohol Depend.* **2019**, *194*, 487–494. [CrossRef]
11. AASLD-IDS. HCV Guidance: Recommendations for Testing, Managing, and Treating Hepatitis C. 2018. Available online: https://www.hcvguidelines.org/ (accessed on 30 September 2018).
12. European Association for the Study of the Liver. EASL recommendations on treatment of Hepatitis C: Final update of the series. *J. Hepatol.* **2020**, *73*, 1170–1218. [CrossRef]
13. Stone, J.; Fraser, H. Incarceration history and risk of HIV and Hepatitis C virus acquisition among people who inject drugs: A systematic review and meta-analysis. *Lancet Infect. Dis.* **2018**, *18*, 1397–1409. [CrossRef]
14. Bruneau, J. Sustained Drug Use Changes After Hepatitis C Screening and Counseling Among Recently Infected Persons Who Inject Drugs: A Longitudinal Study. *Clin. Infect. Dis.* **2014**, *58*, 755–761. [CrossRef]
15. Platt, L. Needle and syringe programmes and opioid substitution therapy for preventing HCV transmission among people who inject drugs: Findings from a Cochrane Review and meta-analysis. *Addiction* **2018**, *113*, 545–563. [CrossRef]
16. Martin, N.K.; Hickman, M. Combination Interventions to Prevent HCV Transmission Among People Who Inject Drugs: Modeling the Impact of Antiviral Treatment, Needle and Syringe Programs, and Opiate Substitution Therapy. *Clin. Infect. Dis.* **2013**, *57*, S39–S45. [CrossRef]
17. Windelinckx, T. C-Buddies: Challenges in the comprehensive approach of Hepatitis C management among people who use drugs in harm reduction setting in Antwerp Belgium. In Proceedings of the 6th International Symposium on Hepatitis Care in Substance Users, Organized by International Network on Hepatitis in Substance Users (INHSU), Jersey City, NY, USA, 6–8 September 2017.
18. Dore, G.J. Elbasvir-Grazoprevir to Treat Hepatitis C Virus Infection in Persons Receiving Opioid Agonist Therapy: A Randomized Trial. *Ann. Intern. Med.* **2016**, *165*, 625–634. [CrossRef]
19. Grebely, J.; Robaeys, G.; Bruggmann, P.; Aghemo, A.; Backmund, M.; Bruneau, J.; Byrne, J.; Dalgard, O.; Feld, J.J.; Hellard, M.; et al. Recommendations for the management of Hepatitis c virus infection among people who inject drugs. *Int. J. Drug Policy* **2015**, *26*, 1028–1038. [CrossRef]
20. Remy, A.-J.; Bouchkira, H. Successful Cascade of Care and Cure HCV in 5382 Drugs Users: How Increase HCV Treatment by Outreach Care, Since Screening to Treatment. *J. Dig. Disord. Diagn.* **2019**, *1*, 27–35. [CrossRef]
21. Verma, S. The Final Frontier: Testing through community needle exchange pharmacies in London. In Proceedings of the International Symposium on Hepatitis Care in Substance Users, Cascais, Portugal, 19–21 September 2018.
22. Saludes, V. Community-based screening of Hepatitis C with a one-step RNA detection algorithm from dried-blood spots: Analysis of key populations in Barcelona, Spain. *J. Viral Hepat.* **2018**, *25*, 236–244. [CrossRef]
23. Peters, L. Decentralised HCV care: The SACC project. In Proceedings of the 5th International Symposium on Hepatitis Care in Substance Users, Organized by International Network on Hepatitis in Substance Users (INHSU), Oslo, Norway, 7 September 2016.
24. Messina, V.; Russo, A. Innovative procedures for micro-elimination of HCV infection in persons who use drugs. *J. Viral Hepat.* **2020**, *27*, 1437–1443. [CrossRef]
25. Molinaro, S.; Resce, G. Barriers to effective management of Hepatitis C virus in people who inject drugs: Evidence from outpatient clinics. *Drug Alcohol Rev.* **2019**, *38*, 644–655. [CrossRef] [PubMed]

26. Foschi, F.G.; Borghi, A. Model of Care for Microelimination of Hepatitis C Virus Infection among People Who Inject Drugs. *J. Clin. Med.* **2021**, *10*, 4001. [CrossRef] [PubMed]
27. Schmidbauer, C.; Schwarz, M. Directly observed therapy at opioid substitution facilities using sofosbuvir/velpatasvir results in excellent SVR12 rates in PWID at high risk for non-adherence to DAA therapy. *PLoS ONE* **2021**, *16*, e0252274. [CrossRef] [PubMed]
28. Loo, N. Real-world observational experience with direct-acting antivirals for Hepatitis C: Baseline resistance, efficacy, and need for long-term surveillance. *Medicine* **2019**, *98*, e16254. [CrossRef]
29. Simmons, B.; Saleem, J. Risk of Late Relapse or Reinfection with Hepatitis C Virus after Achieving a Sustained Virological Response: A Systematic Review and Meta-analysis. *Clin. Infect. Dis.* **2016**, *62*, 683–694. [CrossRef]

MDPI
St. Alban-Anlage 66
4052 Basel
Switzerland
Tel. +41 61 683 77 34
Fax +41 61 302 89 18
www.mdpi.com

Journal of Clinical Medicine Editorial Office
E-mail: jcm@mdpi.com
www.mdpi.com/journal/jcm

www.ingramcontent.com/pod-product-compliance
Lightning Source LLC
LaVergne TN
LVHW070545100526
838202LV00012B/382